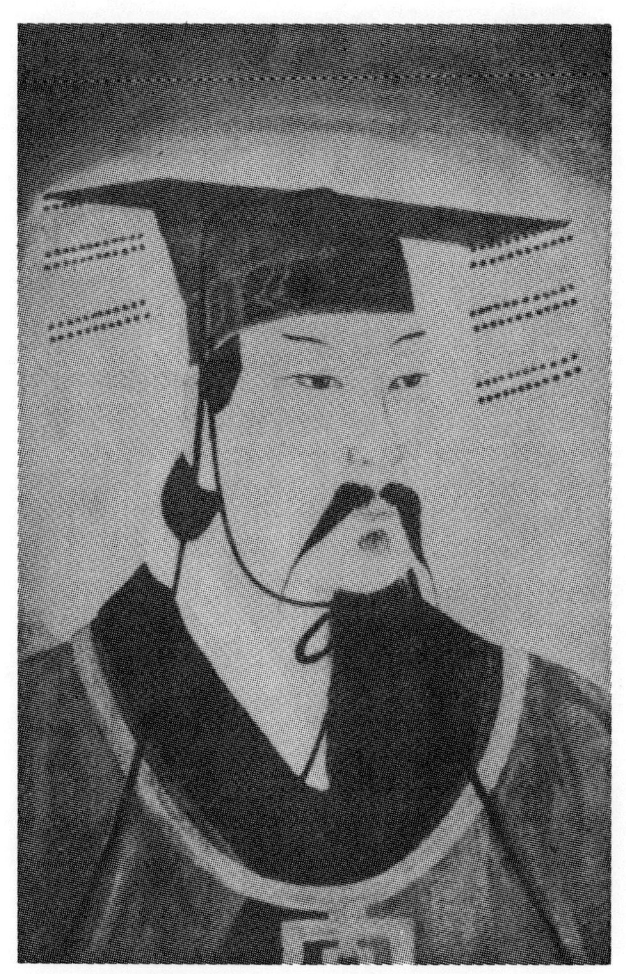

Yellow Emperor

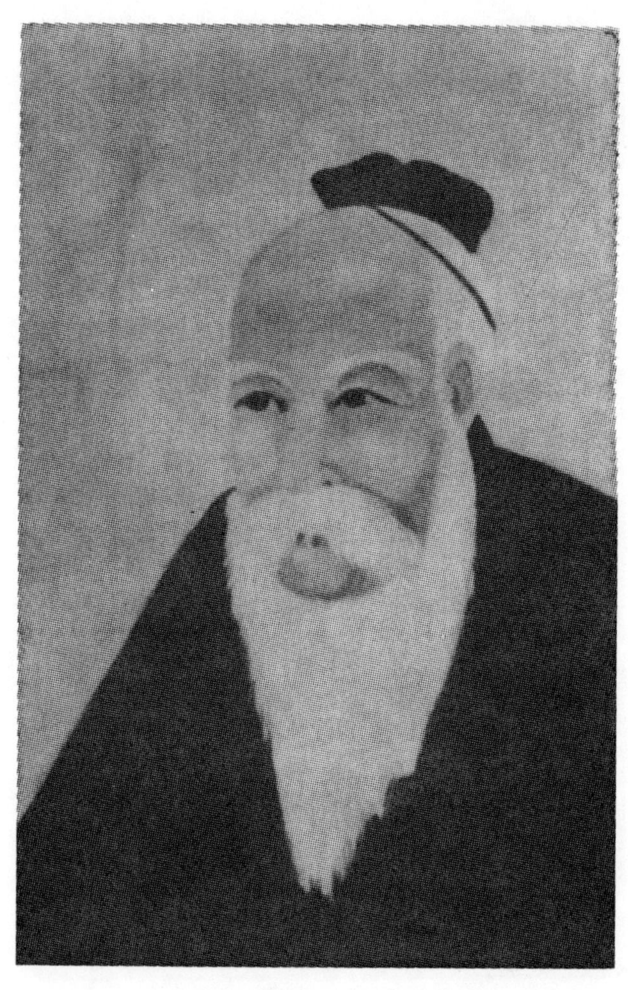

Lao-Tse

THE COMPLETE SYSTEM OF SELF-HEALING

INTERNAL EXERCISES

By Dr. Stephen T. Chang

Tao Publishing

Published by Tao Publishing
2700 Ocean Avenue,
San Francisco, CA 94132

ELEVENTH PRINTING 1995

Printed in the United States of America
Typesetting by Diana Clardy of H.S. Dakin Co., San Francisco

Library of Congress Cataloging in Publication Data

Chang, Stephen Thomas
The complete system of self-healing.

Includes index.
1. Exercise therapy. 2. Medicine, Chinese.
I. Title.
RM725.C438 1986 615.8'2 86-1859
ISBN 0-942196-06-6

Acknowledgements

The author gratefully acknowledges the support and help of:

Vera Brown
Helene Chang
Shirley Dahn
Mako Hayamizu
Sam Matthew
Ed McLean
Rick Miller
Bjorn Overbye, M.D.
Grace Roessler, Ph.D.
Cecilia Rosenfeld, M.D.
Eugene Schwartz
Leonard Worthington, J.D.

About the Author

Stephen Thomas Chang is an internationally well-known scholar. His grandmother was a master-physician, while her father was both personal physician to Empress Tse-Shi and the first Chinese ambassador to the United Kingdom. Dr. Chang has been trained in both Chinese and Western medicine, and in addition to his medical doctor degree, he holds doctor degrees in law, philosophy, and theology. He lectures world-wide on various aspects of Taoism, and he is the founder of the Foundation of Tao. He is also the author of:

The Complete Book of Acupuncture,
The Great Tao,
The Tao of Sexology,
The Tao of Management,
and
The Tao of Healing Diet: Secrets of a Thin Body.

Several books have been translated into ten languages.

Foreword

I would like to take this opportunity to thank every one of the honorable readers throughout the world who has purchased my books since 1978. I greatly appreciate the continuous support, which has been reinforced by thousands of letters of appreciation and inquiry. In regard to these letters, I would also like to take this chance to apologize to those whose letters I have not had a chance to answer. For these people, and others who wish to know more, I have written another book that will answer the many questions and satisfy the many appetites for knowledge. To let the reader know about the supplementations of a great many more healing techniques and new concepts and corrections to the old text, I have changed the title from *The Book of Internal Exercises* to *The Complete System of Self-Healing*. Instead of showing only one room, the new book opens the door to the entire house. I have devoted forty years of intensive research, experience, and meticulous selection to make sure that the techniques within this book are:

★ Absolutely true Taoist teachings (such as the principle of mind and body unification).

★ Absolutely scientific.

★ Proven to possess great healing value.

★ Absolutely natural (equipment, which causes bodily imbalances, is not needed).

★ Absolutely safe (no side-effects) and free from time or space limitations.

I hope you will enjoy this book more, gain more riches in health and knowledge from it, and help more of those who are suffering with the aid of it.

Stephen T. Chang

An Important Note To The Reader

This book was written only to introduce the Internal Exercises of Taoism as a gesture of goodwill. Since certain exercises, special techniques, and teachings which are introduced may be new to certain societies, since human beings are complicated and delicate in constitution, and since every individual is different, please consult your physician before you try any of the contents of this book, for your own protection.

The author and the publisher specifically disclaim liability for any loss or risk incurred by the use or application of any of the contents of this book.

Table of Contents

Introduction

We spend our lives fulfilling two basic physical needs to maintain, nourish, revitalize, and prolong our lives. These are:

1. Consumption (eating, drinking, etc.)
2. Motion
   a. Mind "movement" (thinking)
   b. Body "movement" (breathing and other functions of the internal organs and external limbs)
   c. Sex

Life will cease if either of the two basic conditions is not fully or properly satisfied. Without consumption of nutrients, life is expected to cease within ten days. Without *proper* consumption of nutrients, life will shorten. Without motion, the body will atrophy. Without *proper* motion, the body will weaken. It was with this last consideration in mind that the ancient Taoists created the Tao of Revitalization, the philosophy and method of thinking, breathing, and moving.

Tao of Revitalization is a system of many mental and physical movements, called Internal Exercises. The Internal Exercises heal and energize the internal organs—the keys to youth, immunity against disease, and true health—through deceleration, smoothness, quietness, precision, naturalness, and an internal emphasis.

The Internal Exercises are the very opposite of external exercises. While external exercises such as football, boxing, gymnastics, weight-lifting, Hatha Yoga, and martial arts may produce an attractive outer figure, they often do so by depleting the energy of the internal organs, thereby causing not only any number of illnesses, but also premature aging. The fatigue, stress, strain, pain, and contortions associated with the external exercises disrupt the delicate organic functions. Since responsibility for the body's regenerative processes and defenses against disease-causing agents lies in the internal organs, disrupting their functions will impair the body's ability to replace old or worn cells and fight off germs and viruses. The internal organs do what thick muscles can not do: protect the body against age and disease. The Internal Exercises, in turn, protect, heal, and energize the organs. And when internal organs are healthy, attractive figures naturally result.

The creator of this system of movements was the Yellow Emperor, who was also a father of Taoism, the science and philosophy of life and longevity. His original, untranslated name for the Tao of Revitalization is Yang Sheng Shu. One can define the latter term as the achievement of a happy, healthy, and long life through the utilization of mental and physical movements to prevent and correct all ailments, reverse the aging process, and improve all functions of the body.

Tao of Revitalization has a six thousand year long history of success. Upon realizing its enormous medicinal potential, the Yellow Emperor gave the Tao of Revitalization the title "The Foremost of Therapies". In the *Tao Te Ching*, Lao-Tse called it the "best therapeutic method for promoting and prolonging life". Its reverent and faithful practitioners are multitudinous. And it was effective even when its expansive teachings were fragmented and disarranged.

Many versions of the Tao of Revitalization exist, each with appropriately descriptive names. These names, however, do not reflect the true meaning and function of the Tao of Revitalization. One version is *Tao-Yin*, which means the utilization of thought, tools, and certain body movements to guide the flow of energy to heal ailments of all kinds. Presently, this version of the Tao of Revitalization is immensely popular in Japan. *Do-in*, as it is called in Japan, is taught in *Do-in* clubs which are organized in every city, village, and neighborhood. Club members meet once or many times a week to help and encourage each other in the practice of selected methods of Do-in, thereby preventing and treating diseases. The form of Tao of Revitalization that is popular in China is *Chi-Kung*, also called *Nei-Kung*. The term *Chi-Kung* translates to Breathing or Energizing Exercises. The term *Nei-Kung* translates to Internal Exercises.

In China, a scientific study was conducted on *Chi-Kung* therapy by Dr. Pao Ling. His work, published in *Guolin Research Report*, involved 2,873 terminal cancer patients who took part in an experiment wherein *Chi-Kung* therapy was used to treat their afflictions. Within a six-month period, about 12% of the patients were cured and about 47% showed significant improvements in their conditions. About 41% showed no improvement. Another experiment involving school children was conducted to test one part of *Chi-Kung*—the eye exercises. Their exercise routine was accompanied by music and instructional intercom announcements. As results of the exercises, farsightedness, nearsightedness, and other eye problems became a rare affliction. Other experiments conducted on *Chi-Kung* therapy demonstrated tremendous and rapid efficaciousness against sinus allergies, hemorrhoids, prostate problems, and aging. In the hospitals, clinics, and health organizations of China, *Chi-Kung* therapy reigns supreme above other treatments, such as chemotherapy, surgery, and acupuncture. Its effectiveness was found to lie in its ability to cure and *prevent* disease.

In the U.S., a scientific study was conducted on the Internal Exercises by Dr. Cecilia Rosenfeld. After practicing the Internal Exercise and experiencing an immediate improvement in health, Dr. Rosenfeld decided to prescribe these exercises to her patients. Internal Exercises were taught to her patients, and within one week, about 80% of the patients showed positive results. Then eight nurses were hired, taught about the Internal Exercises, and trained in the instruction and supervision of patients. Afterward, several patients were assigned to each nurse after the patients were examined and given a prescription of specific Internal Exercises. Most patients reported that they experienced immediate improvements in health, without feeling pain or discomfort, and the nurses themselves reported that they had boundless energy even after a day of performing and demonstrating the exercises. As one nurse explains: "It used to be that a nurse's life was miserable. Every day all we saw was sickness, suffering, pain, and death. We heard only complaints. The patients never called the nurse to say 'Isn't it a nice day?' After working eight hours on our feet, we felt as if we were ready to die. But now, since we started using these exercises—a hundred times a day—we feel as if we're ready to jump through the roof at the end of the day! We have so much energy we can't stand it anymore!"

As a result of this study, the Internal Exercises became a subject of study for many universities, colleges, medical schools, hospitals, and the general public.

What underlies such miraculous results?

Prevention, a principle of the Tao of Revitalization, is one key to the

Internal Exercises' efficacy: if minor health problems do not develop, major health problems do not develop, and if major health problems do not develop, we will not die. So the primary purpose of Tao of Revitalization is to help people increase their lifespan.

Therefore, Tao of Revitalization is not a sport. It is not designed to provoke competition and strenuous movements, increase stress or tension, deplete energy, or, in other words, decrease one's lifespan. Neither is it a form of martial art. Unlike Kung Fu, Karate, etc., it involves neither strenuous movements nor tension. Although the movements in T'ai Chi Chuan appear slow, they actually build tension, for T'ai Chi Chuan was originally designed for combat. However, one aspect of T'ai Chi Chuan, that of the unification of mind and body, is similar to that of the Tao of Revitalization. Further, Tao of Revitalization is not Hatha Yoga in that it does not overwhelm the body with a series of twisting, bending, or stretching poses and motions. Lastly, Tao of Revitalization is not another form of meditation, because the objective of the most popular forms of meditation is to "empty" the mind—inactivate the mind. The mind cannot be emptied, for directing it to do so is itself an activation of the mind.

In the Tao of Revitalization, the emphasis has been lifted to internal, rather than external, development. Initially the Tao of Revitalization involves physical movement, but as one's practice gradually becomes refined, one's concentration upon physical movement will be reduced and one's concentration upon internal movement will be increased. One will become still externally, but alive and active internally. Anything that does not meet these principles is not Tao of Revitalization.

Its strength also lies in Tao of Revitalization's flexibility. Anybody, regardless of age, health, or condition, can practice the exercises of his or her choice anytime, anywhere. No equipment is necessary. The most basic of metabolic processes, breathing, can be transformed by the appropriate Tao of Revitalization techniques into a powerful therapy. The conscious state of mind and body movement are also potential therapies.

The heartwarming benefits so immediately reaped from a sincere and selfless application of any of the exercises are enough to instill within us a kind of fervor which of itself will move us forward along the path of greater understanding, longevity, and spiritual development.

When you do external exercises,
you must do internal exercises.
When you do internal exercises,
you may forget to do external exercises.

PART I

UNDERLYING PRINCIPLES

1

Taoism

The Complete System of Self-Healing: Internal Exercises is about one part of the living philosophy of Taoism. Taoism is the eldest of the world's religions. Its founder, Lao-Tse, the best-known and perhaps greatest of Taoist sages, laid the groundwork which was to support the Eight Pillars of Taoism when he wrote the *Tao Te Ching*. The *Tao Te Ching* itself is primarily a political treatise and a theoretical representation of Taoism expressed from the point of view of an enlightened being. The formulation of the practical and functional aspects was left to other Taoist sages—the Yellow Emperor, for instance. When other ancient Taoist masters devised—in addition to the basic spiritual doctrines and philosophy of Taoism—innumerable techniques designed to ultimately transform and immortalize the physical body, the Eight Pillars of Taoism materialized. The Eight Pillars are eight branches of Taoist thought and practice, and they are symbolized as eight trigrams in the *Pa-Kua*, the symbol of Taoism. The Internal Exercises themselves form one pillar of Taoism.

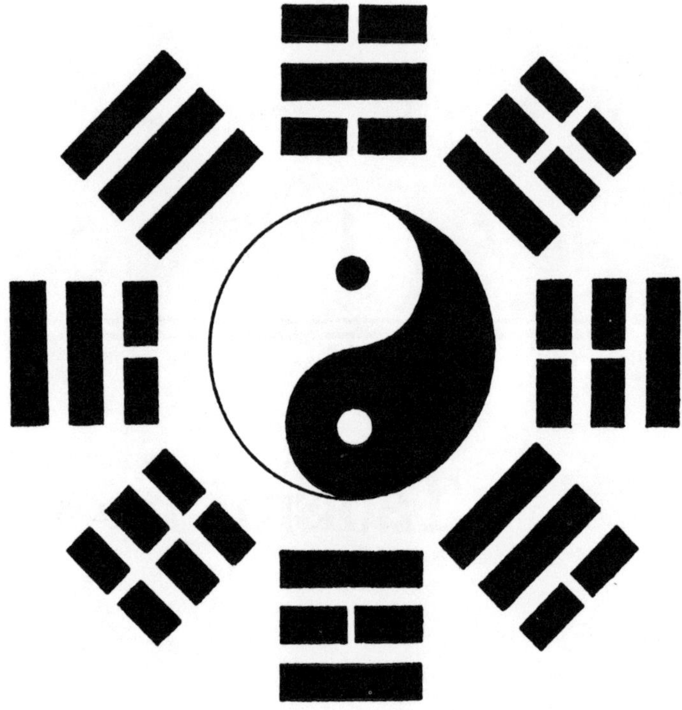

Figure 1. Pa-Kua (Symbol of Taoism). The eight trigrams (pointing in 8 different directions from the Yin-Yang symbol) represent The Eight Pillars of Taoism.

Many true Taoist teachings have been kept secret for many centuries, so before we begin examining the Internal Exercises in detail, the Eight Pillars will be listed and then briefly summarized.

1. The Tao of Philosophy
2. The Tao of Revitalization (Internal Exercises)
3. The Tao of Balanced Diet
4. The Tao of Forgotten Food Diet
5. The Tao of Healing Art
6. The Tao of Sex Wisdom
7. The Tao of Mastery
8. The Tao of Success

THE TAO OF PHILOSOPHY

The Tao of Philosophy discloses the logic underlying the way life unfolds and the purpose of destiny. It is a collection of guidelines that is used by the individual as well as the collectivity for attaining success and spiritual elevation. Based on the spiritual discovery of hidden but ever-permeating and reliable laws of this universe, the Tao of Philosophy provides detailed information on the proper methods of government and fosterage of social development and individual well-being.

THE TAO OF REVITALIZATION

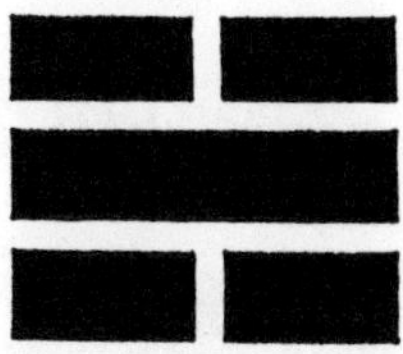

This is the subject of this book, the purpose of which is to explain clearly the complete theory and practice of the Tao of Revitalization.

The Internal Exercises direct the innate healing power to specific internal organs and glands to energize the entire body, balance the energy level, and promote a more effective functioning of the internal organs, in order to heal, adjust, correct, and above all prevent disease. In sum, their main purpose is to promote longevity.

There are three categories of Internal Exercises.

The first category of Internal Exercises includes those designed to correct sitting, reclining, walking, and working postures, to facilitate healing. These exercises are the Five Animal Exercises, Eight Directional Exercises, Twelve Zodiac Exercises, and Twelve Nerve Exercises. Also included are the basic exercises known as the Deer Exercise, the Crane Exercise, and the Turtle Exercise.

The second category includes Meridian Meditation, also known as Trip-Around-the-World Meditation, or simply Taoist Contemplation. A tremendous healing art, Meridian Meditation is used to adjust, balance, and elevate the energy level in the body. By meditating on the pathways of energy in the body, anatomically known as the meridians, a person is able to feel the energy flow along these pathways and balance the energies within the body. The mind, body, and spirit are completely integrated, and the individual is completely enlivened.

Acupuncture and acupressure techniques, which originated from Meridian Meditation, are used to help others, whereas Meridian Meditation is used to heal oneself.

The third category of Internal Exercises concerns energy breathing techniques. Through these techniques, energy can be absorbed through the acupuncture points which lie atop the meridians which traverse the body. Energy breathing is a vital step in self-healing and in forming an indivisible link with the energy permeating the universe.

THE TAO OF BALANCED DIET

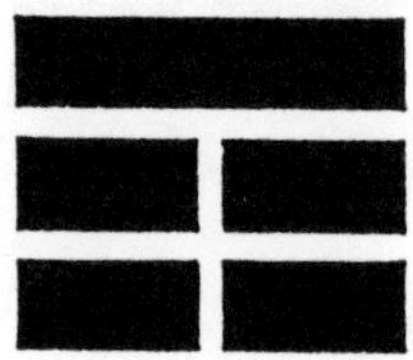

The acid-alkaline balance of our food is very important. Foods that are pH-balanced will not corrupt quickly, and the eater will be able to extract the maximum amount of nutrition available from those foods. If the food we eat is not pH-balanced, it becomes corrupt as soon as it enters the digestive tract. The body, instead of benefiting from the nutrients in the food, absorbs the poisons resulting from the corruption. (If one ever goes to the back door of any restaurant, one will find food corrupting in garbage cans. Not long ago, this food was served to customers. So the only thing separating the front and back of the restaurant is a wall and a few hours' time.) We would not purposely eat garbage because we know we will become sick from ingesting its poisons. Yet, we do eat garbage every time we eat without a thought for pH balance. (A telltale sign of food corruption in the stomach is bad breath.) For a complete study of the Tao of Balanced Diet, please refer to the *Tao of Healing Diet: Secrets of a Thin Body*.

THE TAO OF FORGOTTEN FOOD DIET

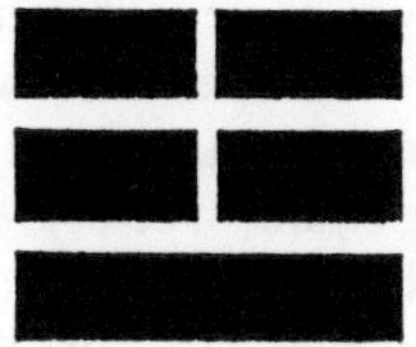

We rely on our regular diet for enjoyment and satisfaction: we take pleasure in the appearance, smell, and taste of our daily meals. But regular foods do not provide enough nutrients to maintain a continuous state of health. They must be supplemented with stronger foods, or herbal foods, which constitute the second level of diet, or Tao of Forgotten Food Diet.

Over the ages, Taoists thoroughly studied the healing composition of herbs and became highly proficient at the use of herbs. For example, several thousand years ago, surgeons were able to anesthetize their patients for six hours without side-effects just by using an herb tea. (Surgery was very popular at that time. The surgeons often removed the organs of the patient, washed them in herbal solutions, and reorganized them inside the body. This practice eventually died out as these doctors came to realize that it was an inefficient and incomplete treatment for illnesses and that the final answer lay in illness prevention. They realized that any illness, including tumors, was the result of a particular lifestyle; constant surgery could not prevent the recurrence of tumors, whereas a change in lifestyle could prevent the recurrence of tumors.)

Herbs have many properties that modern science has yet to discover. The Academy of Sciences currently estimates that there are approximately one million plant varieties in the world. As yet, only an insignificant portion has been examined by modern means of analysis.

The food we buy in the supermarket is the weakest food available. The selection there is very limited if one considers the varieties of food actually available in the world. God created leaves, branches, trunks, and roots for our consumption, but they were completely overlooked by most people. Called "forgotten foods" by Taoists, herbs were forgotten because they were eliminated from our ancestors' diets through a process of selection which, over the course of thousands of years, rejected foods that were unappealing to the eyes, nose, or mouth. When man learned to cultivate his own food, he naturally chose to cultivate only those foods that appealed to his senses. As the saying goes, we are what we eat. If we eat stronger foods, we become stronger ourselves. If we eat better foods, our health improves. But, if we eat weak foods, we become more vulnerable to diseases. When we compare a magnolia tree to a bunch of celery, we will see that the tree is much stronger than the little clump of celery. Investigating further, we will find that the tree is of greater medicinal value than the celery. In fact, the various properties of the magnolia tree build up the stomach tissues and strengthen the female sexual organs. Ginseng is another example of a strong food. It grows in cold and harsh mountainous regions, yet it can survive for more than a thousand years. Imagine what such great vitality could do for your body. (Please use discretion when ingesting ginseng. It must be balanced with other herbs, since it produces strong side-effects as well as benefits.) In sharp contrast, a carrot grows only in temperate climates and its lifespan is about three months. If you do not unearth it within three months, it will decay and disappear. Herbs give everlasting strength, whereas regular foods give only temporary strength.

The foods we commonly eat and love are also eaten and loved by the germs in our bodies. They utilize this food (organic or junk) to maintain their lives just as we do. Fortunately, herbs do not nourish germs and human beings equally. Human beings, exercising their will power, are able to ingest sometimes distasteful herbs. Germs, not being blessed with will power, are simply repelled by herbs. When human blood is permeated with herbal nutrients, the germs in the body will starve to death, and the human body will be naturally cleansed and purified. The cleansing and purifying qualities that allow herbs to last for years without rotting are the greatest benefits to be gained from herbal diets.

THE TAO OF HEALING ART

Like the Tao of Revitalization, the Tao of Healing Art adjusts, balances and elevates vital energy. Unlike the Tao of Revitalization, which is primarily a means for self-healing, the Tao of Healing Art is utilized for healing others.

The Tao of Healing Art, also called Tui-Na, is basically a form of massage that follows the body's energy pathways, anatomically known as meridians, to regulate the body's vital functions. By using the sixteen different handling or manipulating techniques of Tui-Na, one can also reposition disarranged internal organs. In conjunction with these techniques, which were designed to adapt to various parts of the body, appropriate mediums can also be used. These can be any of the five fundamental elements: earth, metal, water, wood, or fire. Acupuncture needles (used to channel energy into the body) and moxibustion are two of the best known metal and fire mediums in the West. Acupuncture and moxibustion are derivations of Tui-Na principles and methods. For more information, please refer to *The Great Tao*, Chapter 5.

THE TAO OF SEX WISDOM

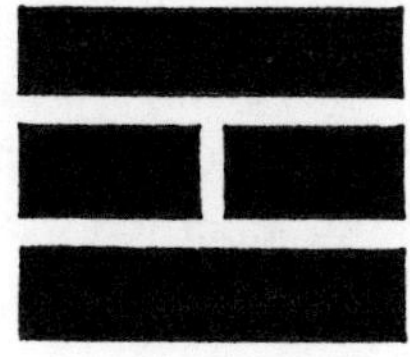

Taoism was the first philosophy to take human sexuality fully into account, to present it in such a way that people could use their sexual energy to transform themselves. Taoist Sexology directs people so they can enjoy sexual play without depleting themselves, explains how to strengthen the sexual organs and use sexual energy to cure specific ailments, strengthens the bond of love, elucidates various positions of therapeutic intercourse, provides natural methods of family planning and eugenics, even includes ways of selecting the sex of your child. For a complete study of The Tao of Sex Wisdom, please refer to the book *The Tao of Sexology.*

THE TAO OF MASTERY

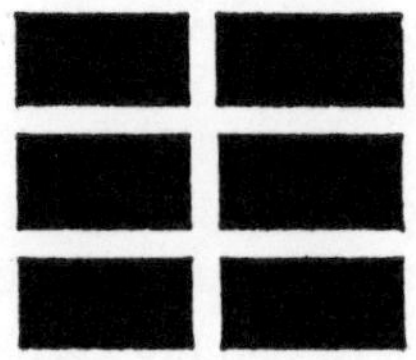

The Tao of Mastery provides us with tools to help us gain insight into ourselves and others, bend surrounding energies to our nature and purpose, and become masters of ourselves.

In order to facilitate personal and working relationships and reduce stress, the ancient Taoists developed a collection of different methods:

1. PERSONOLOGY reveals the current abilities, attitudes, personal traits, and health conditions of an individual. Instinctive anticipation of forthcoming events is reflected in some of the 108 locations of the face, constituting a recognizable warning system.

2. FINGERPRINT SYSTEM reveals the inherited part of personality and health tendencies. Also, fingerprints are changing delineations of our naturally developing personal and professional potentials and are warning signals of our inherited weaknesses, which we must be aware of in order to conquer them.

3. TAOIST NUMEROLOGY gives precise insights into our life patterns and circumstances.

4. NORTH STAR ASTROLOGICAL SYSTEM—more comprehensive and scientific than Western astrology—reveals our destinies and financial prospects; describes the physical, mental, and spiritual attributes of our spouse and children; and unveils all other facets of our lives.

5. DIRECTIONOLOGY is the study of the surrounding physical laws of nature, especially those of electromagnetism. A complete knowledge of such forces allows us to orient ourselves and our belongings in ways compatible with the electromagnetic influences, in order to live in harmony with the laws of nature and facilitate obtainment of goals. On the collective level, it can be used to reduce in-fighting and promote the "chemistry" or cooperation between workers. It is used in modern Japan to organize working groups as well as coordinate the various departments of a company. In the West, the awareness of these influences is reflected in conversations about the "ambience" or the "morale" at working places.

6. SYMBOLOGY deals with forms and symbols related to the laws underlying natural events. It can be used to condition, for instance, weather changes, business trends, self-defeating habits, etc.

THE TAO OF SUCCESS

The Tao of Success discloses the precise mechanics of life's greatest events and the forces that shape all events. The ancient Taoists discovered analytical methods to study these forces, identified recognizable patterns of change, and systematized strategies of success to deal with these patterns. The Tao of Success helps you adjust your everyday actions in accordance with the universal law, to make every aspect of life more pleasant.

A clear and powerful instrument of Taoist wisdom, the Tao of Success is divided into three parts:

1. The study of symbols and signs that represent the endless changes that occur throughout the universe. These phenomena are governed by exact laws defined by physics, chemistry, biology, geometry, algebra, and other branches of mathematics.

2. The Tao of Change, or the study of social philosophy and transactional psychology, as represented by sixty-four hexagrams. Each hexagram is composed of six lines, each of which represents a developing stage in individual or group transactions. Recognition of a certain pattern allows one to develop successful, detailed, and accurate strategies against the causes of adversity. The Tao of Change is invaluable to those who wish to develop wealth, power, harmonious familial relations, social position, and foresight fully.

3. The actual practice of forecasting events, known as the Space and Time I-Ching System. This system is based on the principle of cyclicalness—that is, everything that has happened is going to happen again, and everything that is going to happen has happened already in some form. Like Albert Einstein, the ancient Taoists understood that time was illusory. Like him, they studied situations in the space-time system. Thus, they arrived at a means for interpreting events occurring within our time concept. This is the key to "forecasting", or seeing into the future.

The Eight Pillars of Taoism cover every aspect of our daily existence. They were designed to completely satisfy our basic physical needs in a manner that allows us to realize our full potential as human beings. Then may we leap beyond the degenerating aspect of time, to live with the Tao, or God.

2

The Energy Theory

The root of the way of life, of birth and change is Chi (energy); the myriad things of heaven and earth all obey this law. Thus Chi in the periphery envelops heaven and earth. Chi in the interior activates them. The source wherefrom the sun, moon, and stars derive their light, the thunder, rain, wind and cloud their being, the four seasons and the myriad things their birth, growth, gathering and storing: all this is brought about by Chi. Man's possession of life is completely dependent upon this Chi.

Nei Ching

The ancient Taoist texts, expounding on the basic theories that energy supported all life and matter in the cosmos, were written to convey basic scientific principles in a style that attracted the attention of even those who were not inclined toward a serious study of science. This is not to imply that the barriers between the artistic, scientific, and practical ways of life were as distinct and offered such a marked degree of specialization as are those characterizing modern civilization. The integrated man, as he existed in ancient China, was one who constantly strove to maintain a balance between the various modes of life—the artistic, the scientific, and the practical. It was no great effort for the scientist to record his observations in a style that today would be called "poetic" in form—it came to him naturally. That scientific principles could be conveyed in such imaginative form attests to the unification of art and science which typifies the Golden Age of Chinese civilization.

It may well be that because the basic principles of Taoism are poetically stated, many modern scientists choose to reject them, avowing them to be "unscientific", "purely philosophical", "mystical", and "primitive". But the rejection of traditional principles on these grounds, far from indicating a greater degree of objective awareness on the part of the modern day men of science, suggests instead a growing gap between science and the true "art of living". The principles of Taoism and the Internal Exercise system as they have come down through the ages are just as applicable today as they were in the past, but they must be interpreted through a proper understanding of the poetic form that has enshrined and carried them through the ages.

THE NATURE OF ENERGY

Energy is a dynamic force, in constant flux, which circulates throughout the body. Many people plausibly substitute the word *life* for the word *energy*, since the essential difference between the two words is so subtle that it eludes all but the semanticist. Each term is vital to developing an accurate understanding of the energy theory as it applies to the body.

For all practical purposes, it can be stated that life is an *indication* of energy within the body. All that comes to mind on hearing the word *life*—breathing, talking, sleeping, eating, even the ability to read, think, and hear—all these can be achieved only because of the energy within the body. This invariably applies to those functions or activities that are not conspicuously perceptible; for example, the metabolic processes within each single cell could not be accomplished without energy to sustain those functions. Energy is the basis for the apparent solid structures of the body and all that pertains to its anatomy. For what is a solid structure such as a bone, except a mass of living cells? All forms and activities of life, both anatomical and physiological, are supported by, and simultaneously deplete, the energy within the body.

Although most people assume that inert matter is completely solid or dense, it is energy that binds the protons, electrons, and neutrons within each individual atom. Inanimate matter, then, is simply energy at a different rate of vibration than that of other forms of life. *Energy therefore is the absolute basis for all forms of life and matter in the universe.*

Food and air are considered to be the primary sources of energy to be depleted through daily living rather than as fuel to be metabolized by the body. Energy, though, is not obtained from the gross molecular aspects of food and air, but rather from what can be called its "vibrational" essence, or, its electromagnetism. For instance, the nutrients within any particular food can be accurately reproduced in a chemist's laboratory, but life cannot be sustained over a prolonged period of time by ingesting those synthetic nutrients alone: it is possible to obtain every single vitamin, mineral, and chemical that comprises an egg, and yet it is impossible to transform them into anything that vaguely resembles a genuine egg. Neither is a person able to exist over a prolonged period of time on pure oxygen which has been obtained by laboratory methods, or in a room in which the air has been filtered by an electrical air-conditioner. In all of these instances something is lacking, and that "something" is the particular object's *life force*, its electromagnetism—that invisible energy which enlivens gross molecular aspects of any object.

Electromagnetism is a force with which most of us are not yet familiar. It was Western scientists who ingeniously verified the existence of electromagnetism, providing thereby a means for the logical explanation for many of the health enhancing benefits obtained through the practice of the Internal Exercises. In short, electromagnetism is an intensity force that permeates the atomic structures of all objects, including the surrounding atmosphere. Because it is a natural force, it has a rapport with the energy within the body. The Internal Exercises are mediums through which energy is channeled from the atmosphere into the body to stimulate the body's natural abilities to replenish the energy depleted through daily living.

ENERGY AND THE HUMAN BODY

The self-perpetuating human body can be considered as a type of battery. The human battery is composed of three vital parts:

1. Structure—the cells and the organs, bones, muscle, skin layers, blood vessels, nerves, and other physical structures that they form.

2. Liquid—the intra- and inter-cellular liquids that play important roles in the generation of electrical energy.

3. Electrical charge—the charge that is responsible for activating the body and its structures. It is called the "life force", "life energy", "spirit", or electromagnetism. Taoists refer to this force as "Chi".

Of the three components, the last—electrical charge—is least understood since its presence is not immediately obvious to the naked eye. Electrical energy is detected only in a roundabout way, because it is most obvious when it is absent. If there is a partial absence of energy in the body, weakness or disease invades and grasps hold of the body. When there is a total absence of vital-energy, there is death. (Cessation of heartbeat does not necessarily mean death, for many yogis have stopped their own heartbeat, yet remain alive because their bodies still hold vital energy.) Exhaustion is a symptom of low energy levels. Anytime you use your body or your mind, you lose energy. If you fix your eyes on an object for just one minute, it will take you twenty minutes of rest to recharge the amount of energy lost, according to scientific studies. Furthermore, studies have been done in which dying people have been put on a scale and weighed. At the point of death, there has been recorded a weight loss of about six ounces, the exact amount varying from individual to individual. So it is apparent that the approximate six ounce weight loss reflects the weight of this vital energy, which is material and measurable.

In one particular instance, however, energy can be seen by the naked eye to emanate from the body and act as an indicator of health. The "aura" or energy field around a person's body has been known for thousands of years, but is only now been proven to exist with the advent of Kirlian photography. It is able to capture the aura in photographs so that many people can see it first hand. A simple description of the aura can be that it is made up of colored "flames" of energy that are emitted from the human body. The colors of the aura have been determined to be reflective of its owner's health and energy level. Light, clear colors indicate good health and high energy levels. Dark, heavy colors indicate disease. The color of death is black.

Minute after minute, hour after hour, day after day we are losing energy as our attention is caught by continuous external objects and activities, as we move our bodies in inefficient ways, or as we use energy in continuous mental activities. In time, through this constant loss of energy, we grow weak and are unable to fight off invasion by germs and other harmful disease-causing agents. Illness drains the body of energy, and without energy, cells and tissues stop regenerating and shrivel and die. So weakness is the first step toward disease. If we have no weakness, then it will be impossible to contract a mild illness, and if we never have a mild illness, then a serious disease will never develop. Of course we also acquire vital energy too, through food, air, and cosmic radiation. But as we grow older, we tend to use more energy than we take in, and this empties our store of energy until a final loss of energy results in death.

Then there is the matter of energy imbalance, the importance of which equals energy loss. Energy imbalance among the organs (functionally interlocked like clockwork) is another source of illness. The energy level within an organ is determined by the vigor and regularity of its pulsations. The normal heart rate is 72-78 beats per minute. If this rate reaches or exceeds 80 beats/minute, a fever or high energy is indicated. The normal pulsation rate of one kidney is 36 pulsations per minute, and because we have two kidneys, the total rate is 72 pulsations/minute. The heart and kidneys are therefore balanced with respect to each other. Now if the person owning these organs takes diuretic pills, that person is forcing more pulsations into the kidneys. What happens to the heart? The heart, in order to maintain balance, pumps faster, and this results in high blood pressure and increased blood flow to the kidneys. Since the kidneys filter urine out of blood, more blood means more work for the kidneys. In taking the diuretic pills, that person has created a vicious cycle between his heart and kidneys. How would this affect the rest of the body? If one cogwheel of an intricate clockwork speeds up, the other cogwheels must also speed up, otherwise all the springs and wheels will jam and bring all activity to a stop. Thus we expose ourselves to grave dangers.

To be totally free of disease, however, does not guarantee a state of physical immortality, for the body must be able to accommodate the influx of additional energy which in the end will transform it into a vehicle unconditioned by space and time.

How can we avoid energy loss and imbalance and their aftereffects and still be able to transform our bodies? Let us examine some methods that may fulfill these conditions.

The first is restful sleep. Normally, the human "battery" recharges itself every night when you sleep. After the day's activities, thoughts, and concentrations have depleted most of your energy, you will feel drowsy and fall asleep, so that your body can recharge itself. Sleep relaxes the meridianal points of entry and exit and allows the energy of the universe to enter all the acupuncture points, travel through all the meridians (to be discussed later), and reach and recharge every cell in your body. The next morning when you awaken, your battery is recharged and your energy level is high again. Like the battery and generator in a car, the human battery recharges automatically—if everything is functioning as it should be. If everything functions excellently, everything takes care of itself and you do not have to do anything. But when you do not sleep well, the natural processes are blocked. Then what do you do?

Another alternative can be acupuncture. Since energy supports all vital functions associated with the body, adjusting that energy with acupuncture regulates those functions supported by that energy. This is achieved because of the antenna-like qualities of the acupuncture needles, which serve to bring more energy into the body and make efficient use of its beneficial properties. (An alternate form of acupuncture, called acupressure because hands are used instead of needles, can be used to achieve similar results.) But acupuncture has a limited range of use. It is effective only when the problem is a lack of energy; any problem related to cell structure or liquids will prove acupuncture useless.

Another alternative, external exercises, would not be the proper solution. As explained before, external exercises hasten the aging process and energy depletion, and they offer no means for recovering the energy lost.

Only the three categories of Internal Exercises meet the dual requirements of preservation and transformation. Through the Internal Exercises, diseases of the body can be eliminated by readjusting the energy imbalance that is the unseen cause of the apparent dysfunction, and self-healing, which is the natural result of doing these exercises on a regular basis, is guaranteed. The ways the Internal Exercises preserve the internal organs to preserve health and youth will gradually unfold in the following chapters, as well as the ways the Internal Exercises generate and utilize the higher order of energy to awaken the spiritual center of the body. By learning the Internal Energizing Exercises we are thus able to gain control over the vast energy upon which life depends. We can then use this energy to heal ourselves as well as others, and insure our continuing health and spiritual growth.

3

The Circulation Theory

The circulatory system of the human anatomy is in many respects a transportation system. Oxygen fixated upon red blood cells in the lungs is transported in the bloodstream to every cell in the body. The wastes eliminated by cells are conveyed through the bloodstream to the excretory system, which excretes the wastes but saves the blood cells for further utilization. Nutrients are also conveyed from the intestine to the cells through the bloodstream.

When circulation of the blood is impeded, the body is besieged by problems. Upon the delay of nutrients or oxygen, cells die from the lack of sustenance. Upon the impediment of blood flow, efficiency of cellular waste elimination is greatly reduced. And upon the accumulation of waste matter due to cellular dysfunction, health problems develop.

This would lead some people to conclude that increasing the rate of circulation will decrease the chances of problems developing inside the body. The method that comes to most people's minds as appropriate for accelerating the circulation is exercise—external exercise. Accelerating the circulation through the acceleration of the heart by external exercise seems logical, when one brings into mind two widely known facts: blood vessels are connected to the heart, and the rate of blood flow is synchronized with the heart rate.

Consequently, an ideal heart rate *during* exercise was determined for different chronological ages. Anyone can determine his or her ideal heart rate by applying the following equation:

220 beats/minute–Number of years (age)=maximum heart rate

The maximum heart rate for a person at forty years of age would be 180 beats/minute (or beats per minute). This is the ideal rate. If that person were to elevate his or her current rate to 80% of the ideal rate during exercise, then that person will be in the normal category. The rates achieved by normal people of different ages are as follows:

Table 1. Maximum Heart Rates During Exercise

Age	*Beats/minute*
20	160
30	156
40	144
50	136
60	128
70	120
80	112

According to the above table, the capacity of the heart deteriorates as age increases. The deterioration increases until the heart ceases to function.

Many exercise books advise that one should try to meet the rates specified in Table 1 for a certain length of time—one hour weekly or more—to maintain good health.

But does forcing the heart to increase its rate really improve the circulation and benefit the heart?

Not necessarily. In the hospital one often sees a patient who suffers from both poor circulation and very high heart rates. Although this person lies in bed with cold hands and feet, his heart beats continuously at 160 beats per minute. These inconsistencies can be explained by the fact that circulation does not depend entirely upon the heart rate, for it is also dependent upon the blood vessels. Artery disease, injury, stress, strain, tension, etc. can block the blood vessel and cause the blood supply to diminish. The body, equipped with fail-safe mechanisms, will respond to the obstruction of the blood vessel by accelerating the heart. However, the supply of blood will remain in a diminished state as the cause of the problem—the blockage—still remains. Not only does the circulation problem remain unresolved, but the heart also is exhausted. At this point we may ask, "If backup efforts to correct poor circulation through heightened heart activity fail, how can further punishment of the heart through exercise be effective?"

Furthermore, the heart also suffers from imbalances in nervous stimulation. The heart is controlled by the the vagus nerve, which lowers the heart rate, and the sympathetic nervous system, which increases the heart rate. The vagus nerve originates in the hindbrain and the sympathetic nervous system originates in the spinal cord. Due to the control of the nerves, the heart pumps involuntarily and continuously from the moment it appears two weeks after conception to the moment death is officially announced. Throughout its lifetime the heart is stimulated more by the sympathetic nervous system than by the vagus nerve. Anger, smoking, coffee drinking, ball-game watching, horror-movie watching, lovemaking, stair climbing, etc. are common causes of the exhaustion of the heart in that they accelerate the heart rate through stimulation of the sympathetic nervous system. If exercise is added to the burdens of the heart, its chances of resting and assimilating nutrients necessary to its tissues are greatly diminished. Then it will fail.

So a better method of improving circulation without adding more burden to the heart is needed.

The Internal Exercises are more than qualified for meeting these needs, as they give total consideration to all factors involved in any ailment. The objective of the many Internal Exercises is different from that of the regular exercises: their main purpose is to relax the entire body so that the afflicted part can receive nourishment and heal itself. Heart exhaustion can be prevented by the utilization of certain Internal Heart Exercises to train or direct the brain to stimulate the vagus nerve (originating in the brain) to lower the heart rate. Local circulation can be improved through utilization of, for example, the Crane Exercise without affecting the heart.

In addition, stress, strain, tension, and hypertension can be relieved through the practice of Meridian Meditation and Crane Exercise (wisdom of the Crane), etc.

Within the past seventeen years in the San Francisco Bay Area, 863 people from my audience have sought help for heart problems and circulatory problems. Their ages ranged from 35 years to 93 years. There were, however, two people who were in their 20's. All of them began practicing Tao of Revitalization instead of ''cardiovascular exercises''. These were the results: 761 individuals led completely healthy lives; 72 individuals did very well after combining their practice with light dosages of medications prescribed by physicians; 27 individuals remained unchanged; 1 individual, a 93-year old lady, died from an accidental fall; another individual, a 56-year old man, died after having two surgeries within five months; and another individual, a 72-year old man, died from a stroke after a family argument.

Many others throughout the world devoutly believe in the Internal Exercises and that they are the best answers for the problems or potential problems of the cardiovascular system.

4

The Seven Glands Theory

The ancient Taoists understood that the human body could not exist unless there was a continuous supply of energy coming into the tissues and organs. They realized that health existed when the energy within the body was balanced and that disease occurred when there was a state of energy depletion or weakness. We receive much of the energy we need from the food we eat and in the air we breathe. However, the body, much like an expensive automobile, must be finely tuned if it is to run properly and utilize this energy to its maximum level. Through the centuries, the seven glands within the body have been understood to be energy centers, responsible for regulating the flow of energy within the various systems in the body. The seven glands, in ascending order within the body, are as follows:

1. The sexual glands—the prostate and testes in the male and the ovaries, uterus, vagina, and breasts in the female—are responsible for hormone secretions, sexual energy and response, and reproduction. The sexual gland is called the "stove" because it is the "fire" or

energy producer for the other six glands. It is called the House of Essence.

2. The adrenal glands—situated on the kidneys—support the functions of the kidneys, bones, bone marrow, and spine. (The drug cortisone destroys the adrenal glands, causing anemia and bone weakening.) The adrenal gland is called the House of Water.

3. The pancreas gland, also called the House of Transcendence, helps maintain control over the entire digestive system, including blood sugar levels and body temperature. If the pancreas is weak and begins to leak its secretions (insulin) into the bloodstream, it will neutralize the blood sugar and cause hypoglycemia, or low blood sugar. A person will then crave food and sweets, which get into the bloodstream, stimulate the pancreas, and cause a further drop in the blood sugar level. After this first stage, diabetes (or hyperglycemia) may follow. Then the pancreas slowly deteriorates. Diabetes causes a person to be dependent on insulin injections, which, while neutralizing the sugar in the blood, do nothing to activate the digestive system. Also, hyperglycemia causes the blood to become thick and heavy, which in turn causes the circulation to become very poor. Then the heart must work harder (people with diabetes usually also have heart problems). Additionally, because all seven glands are interconnected, an improperly functioning pancreas causes the adrenal glands to go out of balance. This imbalance in turn affects the sex glands and kidneys.

4. The thymus gland governs the heart and circulatory system. Its condition can be ascertained by pressing a point midway between the two nipples. If the point is tender, the thymus is not functioning normally and circulation will be abnormal. This gland is also called the House of Heart.

5. The thyroid gland, which maintains the metabolism of the cells in the body, governs growth. It is also associated with the respiratory system. The gland is called the House of Growth.

6. The pituitary gland, or House of Intelligence, governs memory, wisdom, intelligence, and thought. It is located at the base of the skull, in the center of what appears to be a small hole or indentation.

7. The pineal gland, or the House of Spirit, directly affects the other

glands through its secretions. Located at the level of the third eye, in the center of the head, it is the psychic and spiritual center of our body. Only human beings have this gland; only human beings worship God and have the desire and need to do so. Intuition and conscience are associated with this gland.

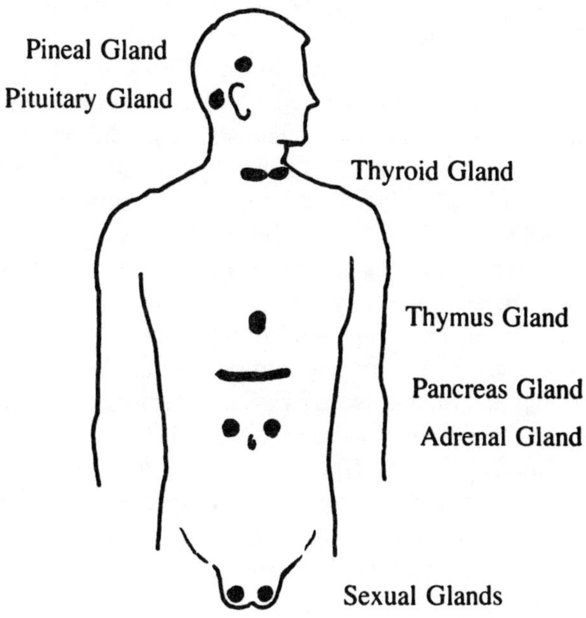

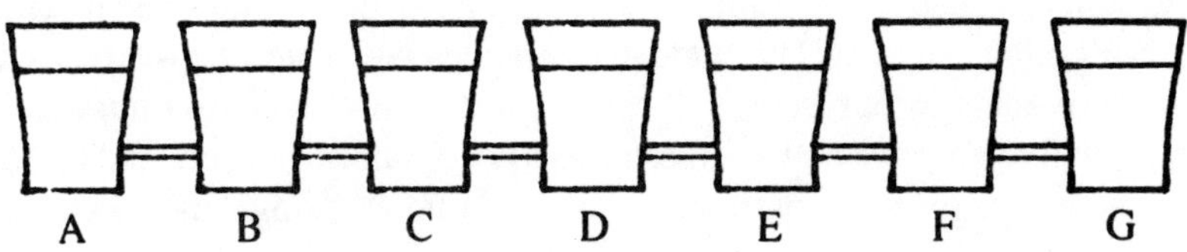

Figures 2a and 2b. The Seven Glands System.

These seven glands may be visualized as vessels that are attached to one another by a series of arteries or tubes. Each vessel (gland) is dependent upon all the others for its supply of liquid (energy). If vessel A (the sexual glands) is supplied with liquid, this fluid will slowly disperse through the arteries to the remaining six vessels. Similarly, if vessel C (the pancreas) were to be drained excessively of its fluid (through a leak of some sort), each of the other vessels would give up a portion of their supply to reestablish an equilibrium within the system. This is similar to how energy flows within our bodies.

(The modern anatomical term for the seven glands is *endocrines*. Endocrinology is a relatively new branch in medical science, and much remains to be discovered by modern scientists. Yet, the ancients have already furnished us with a great deal of information about the structure, nature, and purpose of the endocrine system and the immune system.)

A state of weakness or susceptibility to disease arises when one system, or in this case a gland, is for some reason deprived of energy. Our task becomes then one of not only reestablishing the balanced flow of energy to overcome this weakness, but of also stimulating the flow of energy, so that we raise the level of energy within our bodies to its maximum.

Balancing and raising the energy to its proper level through the Seven Glands System with the Internal Exercises is the Taoist way of strengthening the immune system. Through this method, we can then reverse our existing weakness and heal ourselves, as well as utilize the higher order of energy to open up our spiritual centers. And it is said that if one has strong sexual glands, one may never grow old.

Dr. Alexis Carrel, a Nobel prize winner, stated that the glands system was a "wheel of life". If the wheel of life turned smoothly, problems would not arise or interfere with the cellular processes, which were perpetual. Dr. Carrel, from his extensive experimentations, concluded that every cell was originally immortal. It was immortal if it were not poisoned by polluted air, lack of oxygen, polluted food, and too much acid in the body. (As acid can destroy even stainless steel, it is not hard to imagine its effects on our bodies. Acids accumulate in our bodies when we eat sweets, as they turn into acids in our bodies. Also, a great deal of acid—enough to last through five hours of active digestive activity—must be produced to digest red meat—especially barbecued meat.) Human beings die because of improper care and poisonings.

Therefore, detoxification is the key to longevity, and Internal Exercises are the keys to strong glandular systems that support detoxification.

The sexual glands form the base of the glandular complex, and they support each other in an ascending order. If the first six glands are not filled to their capacity, then the seventh or spiritual house will not be filled either. We may quickly realize that if one were to surgically remove one of the glandular systems, there would be a permanent depletion or disequilibrium within the body. This is why, within the Taoist system of disease prevention, all available routes are explored before surgery is performed, especially if it involves the sexual glands (hysterectomy or prostatectomy), as these comprise the basic foundation that supports all the rest. (In Western medicine, the seven glands are viewed as individual and independent, and are therefore separable. In Taoism, cutting out a gland is viewed as a crime, since doing so would throw the entire body out of balance and open a Pandora's box of health problems. Furthermore, cutting out a part of the body when it is inflamed is like removing a fire detector because one does not like to hear it ring every time there is a fire. The tonsils, the front line of defense for our bodies, are just such a warning system. Because they are attacked by germs first and become inflamed, they are surgically removed, permanently terminating their services as warning systems.) In such a case as the removal of a gland, however, the Internal Exercises would still be important in providing a continued supply of energy and hormones to the body, to prevent the body from weakening further.

The specific Internal Exercises for these purposes would be the Deer Exercise, Dragon Exercise, and one of the Twelve Zodiac Exercises. The Deer Exercise serves to build up the sexual energy ("fire") which then supplies the rest of the glands and body with energy (heat). The Dragon Exercise serves to alleviate imbalanced functioning of these glands. The Zodiac Exercise serves to recharge these glands with the electrical energy of the universe, or electromagnetism.

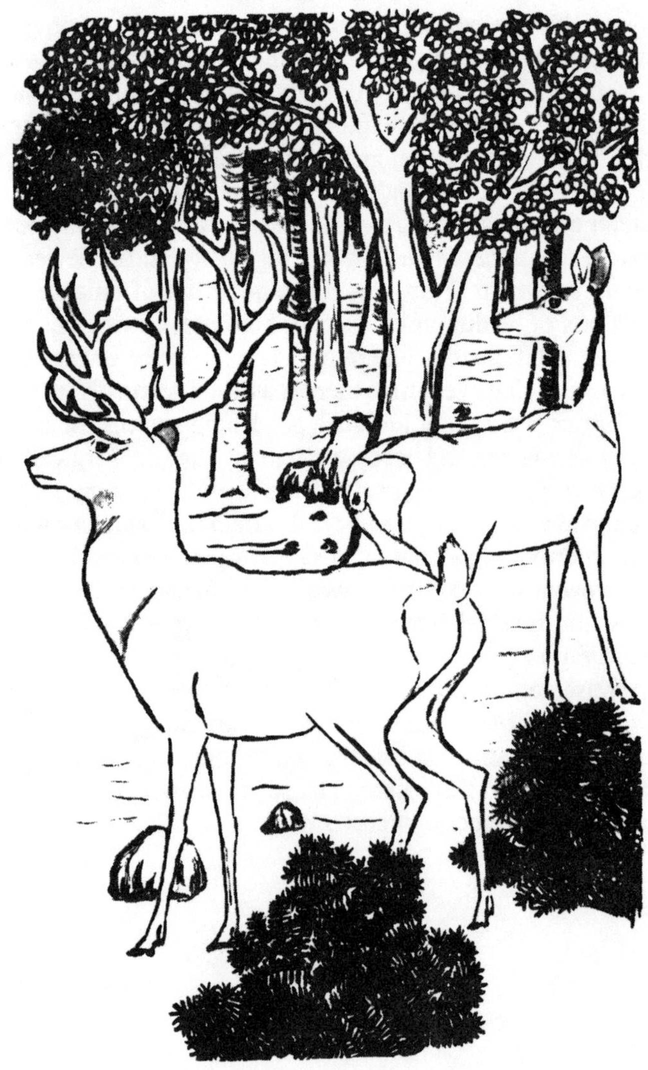

Illustration 1. The Deer.

5

The Nerve Theory

The brain, spinal cord, and nerves are all important parts of the nervous system. According to Taoist theory, many people develop nerve weaknesses because of toxins in their environment and in their food. These toxins accumulate in the liver and the nerves, placing an unnecessary stress on them. This strain weakens the nerves and causes mental imbalance and mental illness, including depression and nervous breakdown. Psychiatric or psychological treatments are not employed by Taoists because they attribute all mental imbalances to nerve weakness, which is a physical imbalance. Taoists believe that once the nervous system is strengthened with the Twelve Nerve Exercises, Crane, Deer and Turtle Exercises, and Liver Exercise, the psychological disturbances will be relieved.

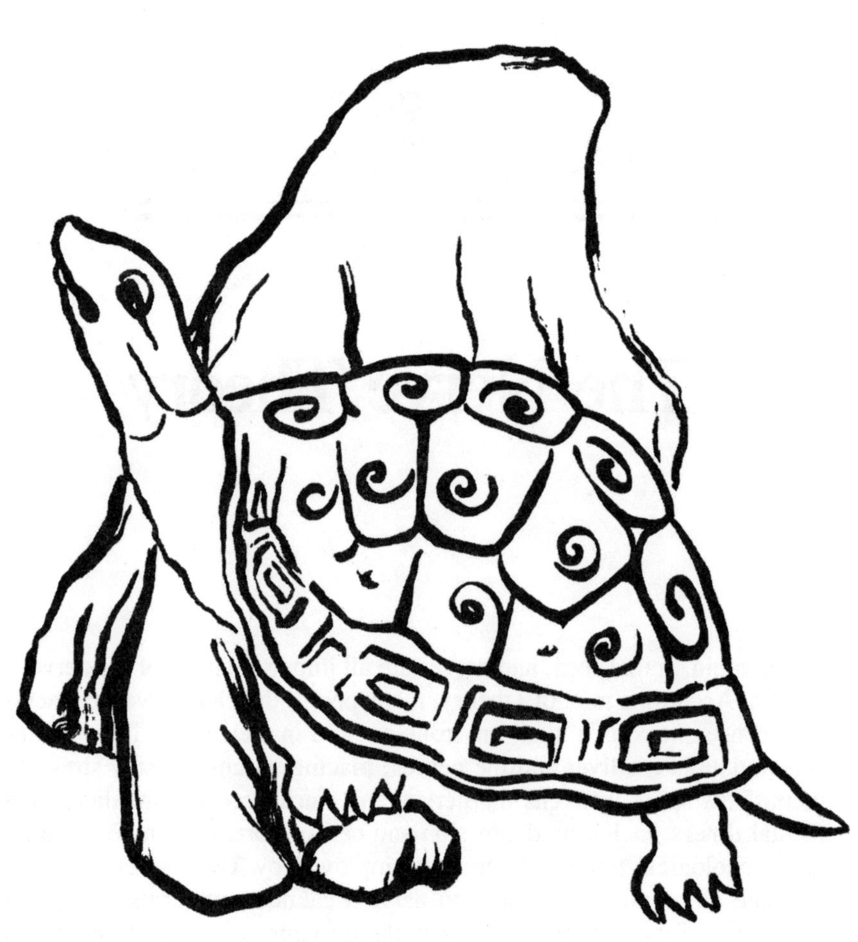

Illustration 2. The Turtle.

PART II

LIVING WITH THE WHOLE BODY

6

The Internal Exercises

The Internal Exercises were arrived at by ancient Taoists through careful study and application of the physical laws of nature and the natural principles of healing. Their conformity to these physical laws—the same laws that govern the human body—confer upon the Internal Exercises the special power to coax the diseased bodily parts back to its natural order, to health. When combined the Internal Exercises make up a wonderful self-healing system that suits every individual's healing needs. When followed daily, they promote not only freedom from disease and pain, but also a wonderful sense of well-being that springs from the heart of the individual. They represent a step which any conscientious person can easily take toward a transformation of the body from the material to the eternal. The Taoists recognized that not everyone would undergo such a transformation during their existing lifetime. However, they emphasized that one still needed to follow these exercises on a daily basis so that one could at the very least obtain perfect health and happiness during one's lifetime. They felt that each man and woman had the right to live a life free of physical pain, mental disharmony, and spiritual selflessness. At a time when most people can only look forward to growing old with a sense of trepidation, this system of Internal Exercises represents an exciting turning point.

Stress—environmental, social, and internal—breeds fear and disease. Presently, growing old conjures up images of high blood pressure, arteriosclerosis, embolisms, cancers, and diseases of all imaginable types. Until recently, westerners have been given few alternatives for dealing with these stresses. We have allowed our bodies and minds to weaken with only cursory hopes of slowing the aging process and preventing disease for a time. However, the main emphasis of the Internal Exercises *is on strengthening our bodies and minds*. They aim to tone all the internal systems, including the emotional and the spiritual. By performing these simple exercises on a daily basis, we can look forward to growing old with a sense of ease and excitement, knowing we carry with us from year to year an inner sense of vitality and alertness which comes only from living a life free from the anxiety of future illnesses and the weakness due to present diseases. Only when we have developed this sense of freedom and this inner vitality will we be able to create a fertile ground upon which our true spiritual nature can unfold. And only then can we attempt to reach out for the transformation of our material bodies into the eternal.

A state of harmony brings with it a feeling that there is no good or bad, positive or negative, Yin or Yang, disease or fear. When a shoulder heals, one often has to be reminded that at one time it suffered great pain. When one reaches this point, it is easy to stop practicing all exercises. Thus one may inadvertently fall back into weakness and disease. One needs, then, an outer sense of discipline at first to continue to pursue this, as is necessary in any endeavor. I hope, however, that an inner sense of discipline will develop within the practitioner to carry him or her forward on a continual movement of interest. This movement arises from the understanding, growth, and feeling of wellness that comes from following these exercises.

The Internal Exercises are easily performed, require no strenuous activity, and do not require a great deal of time to perform. They are a gift to the world from the ancient Taoists, and when used wisely and with a feeling of appreciation, will be well worth the time and energy invested in practicing them. They have been developed around natural laws of healing, and therefore one need not be in a hurry to "master" them. Take your time in developing a feeling for each exercise and you will be rewarded with ample treasures.

The proper use of imagination plays an important part in some of the Internal Exercises. It has been recognized for centuries that a thought is as much a reality as a material object, and in fact, that they are one and the same. They are both forms of energy, the distinguishing difference being that they exist at different frequencies and wave lengths of vibration. Imagination is used, in some cases, to bring together the mind and the body so that they function as a unit. By using our imagination, we may begin to explore our minds and bodies through the Internal Exercises, and in time we will discover extraordinary levels of health existing within us.

The ancient progression set down centuries ago for practicing the Internal Energizing Exercises will be closely followed. One begins with the Five Animal Exercises, the Eight Directional Exercises and the Twelve Zodiac Exercises, and proceeds with the other exercises which work to heal the internal and external systems of the body. Once these initial exercises are mastered, one goes on to the meditative and breathing techniques. The special prescriptions for healing may be used whenever necessary. One may achieve proficiency and freedom from many previous weaknesses and diseases within three to six months after beginning to practice the initial exercises. Proficiency in the meditative and breathing techniques may take longer. Benefits accrue throughout the process however, and this allows us to observe their movement from time to time. We hope the growing sense of vitality and wellness which you feel upon following these exercises will be sufficient to keep you on the path toward physical, mental, and spiritual enrichment.

FIVE ELEMENT THEORY

The ancient Taoists, by observing and contemplating the workings of the universe, devised a theory to explain the balance of the complimentary and antagonistic units of which it is composed. The characteristics and relationships of these dynamic units are explained in the Five Element Theory.

In this theory, the life force in all of its myriad manifestations comes into and goes out of existence through the interplay of five elements: fire, earth, metal, water, and wood. This five-element model is unique to Taoism, because ancient Western and Indian philosophy used a four-element model, which consists of the elements earth, air, water, and fire. In Taoism, air is included in the concept of fire, for without air, fire would not burn.

There are two cycles that illustrate the interaction between these elements. In the first cycle—the cycle of generation—each element generates or produces the succeeding element: wood produces fire, fire produces earth, earth produces metal, metal produces water, water produces wood—the cycle begins again. In the second cycle—the cycle of destruction—each element destroys or absorbs the succeeding element: fire destroys metal, metal destroys wood, wood absorbs water, water absorbs fire, fire destroys metal—the cycle begins again.

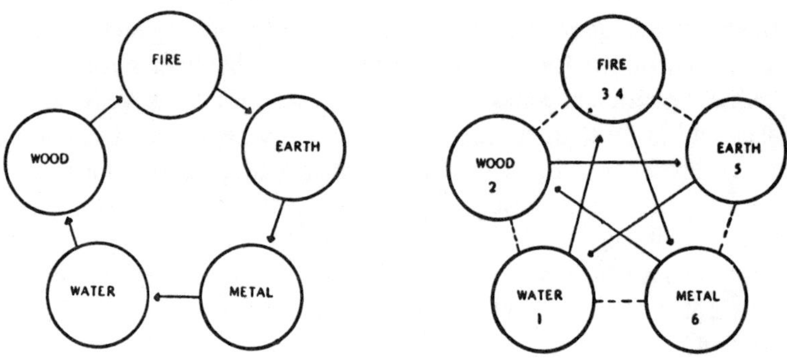

Figure 3. Cycle of Generation. Figure 4. Cycle of Destruction.

Because the universe maintains balance through the interplay of the five elements, our bodies, a microcosm of the universe, are thought to achieve mental and physical harmony in the same way. Energy flows through the body via the meridians and their respective organs and bowels in well-defined cycles. The cycles depicting the flow of energy within the body mirror the two cycles which depict the interaction between the five elements. Taoism identifies each of the viscera with one of the elements in the following manner:

Table 2. The Elements as Assigned to the Organs and Bowels.

Fire—heart small intestine Triple Heater (endocrines) Heart Constrictor (blood vessels)	Metal—lungs large intestine skin
	Water—kidneys bladder bones
Earth—spleen-pancreas stomach muscle	Wood—liver gallbladder nerves

Identifying each of the organs with its respective element in the first cycle results in: the heart (fire) supporting the spleen-pancreas (earth), the spleen-pancreas (earth) supporting the lungs (metal), the lungs (metal) supporting the kidneys (water), the kidneys (water) supporting the liver (wood), and the liver (wood) supporting the heart (fire). The bowels also follow the same cycle: the small intestine (fire) supports the stomach (earth), the stomach (earth) supports the large intestine (metal), the large intestine (metal) supports the bladder (water), and the bladder (water) supports the gallbladder (wood).

If the energy within an organ is not balanced, that organ, rather than being able to effectively support the organ succeeding it on the meridian circuit, will adversely affect, or will be adversely affected by, another organ. This pattern has been depicted in the second cycle of interaction between the elements in which each element destroys or absorbs the other. Thus, when the energy within the heart (fire) is imbalanced, it (heart, fire) will adversely affect the lungs (metal); the lungs (metal) will adversely affect the liver (wood); the liver (wood), the spleen-pancreas (earth); the spleen-pancreas (earth), the kidneys (water); and the kidneys (water), the heart (fire). This pattern also applies to the bowels: imbalanced energy within the small intestine (fire) will cause it to adversely affect the large intestine (metal); the large intestine (metal), the gallbladder (wood); the gallbladder (wood), the stomach (earth); the stomach (earth), the bladder (water); and the bladder (water), the small intestine (fire).

In showing that the cyclic interaction between the organs and bowels is identical to the interaction between the elements, the Taoists not only provided a means by which the sayings, "That which is above is the same as that which is below" and "The microcosm reflects the macrocosm," can be realized and understood, but they also provided a means whereby the interaction of energy between the organs and bowels can be accepted as fact, in that the basis for that interaction is founded upon the very same logic whereby the interaction of the five elements is instinctively realized to be true.

THE FIVE ANIMAL EXERCISES

Taoists modeled five exercises after five animals whose movements were proven effective for the healing of human beings. They were the dragon, tiger, bear, eagle, and monkey. By imitating their characteristic movements human beings can alleviate the imbalanced functioning of their organs, specifically, the five major organs and their related minor organs. That is possible because the movements of a particular animal stimulate a particular five-element organ.

For anyone who is basically healthy, any of the Five Animal Exercises can be used whenever circumstances permit to maintain a balanced physical and emotional state. If a specific problem exists, then one may choose the exercise that deals with the affected organ group or apply what in Taoism is called the Mother and Child Law.

The Mother and Child Law, as it applies to the human body, is based upon the interaction between the five elements. Each element is the "mother" of the succeeding element and, at the same time, the "child" of the element that precedes it in the cycle depicting the flow of energy throughout the elements. For instance, earth is the mother of metal and also the child of fire.

As energy circulates throughout the body, it passes through each organ and bowel in a well-defined cycle. Each organ or bowel is the "mother" of the organ or bowel succeeding it on the circuit; this phenomenon is based on the Five Element Theory. For example, the lungs support the kidneys and therefore the lungs are said to be the "mother" of the kidneys. If the energy within the kidneys (child) is deficient, stimulating the energy within the lungs (mother) with the Eagle Exercise results in an automatic increase of energy in the kidneys, according to the Mother and Child Law. Here, one is treating two organs with one exercise. By consulting the diagram of influences (figures 3 and 4) and Table 2, an exercise or a group of exercises can be selected to suit any need.

In addition to healing and balancing the organs, these exercises also effectively remove tension, stress, anger, and anxiety. According to Taoist theories, stress and tension are the most corrosive enemies of health. Taoists believe that all health problems can be traced to stress and tension, because, even with the best foods and medications, stress and tension can so restrict the functions of the organs that none of the nutrients necessary for cell repair, regeneration, or health can be absorbed.

The proper use of imagination plays an important part in each of the Five Animal Exercises. It has been recognized for centuries that a thought is as much a reality as a material object, and in fact, that they are one and the same. They are both forms of energy. These ancient theories have been confirmed by the work of Dr. Karl Pribram, a Stanford University neurosurgeon and psychologist. Imagination is used, then, to bring together the mind and the body so that they function as a unit. Unifying the image of a particular animal with that of one's body strengthens a person psychologically and physically.

When one performs the exercises, one's thoughts must be fixed upon the image of the animals. The exercise must stop the moment the mind wanders. Also, the miming of the animals' movements must be executed in a free flowing manner.

Never overdo one exercise. If one concentrates too much on the Eagle Exercise (metal), for example, one could decrease the liver function (wood). If you become too relaxed, the nerves will become dulled. But if the liver is overactive—having an augmented energy level—it could be calmed by the Eagle Exercise. So, the key word here is balance.

THE DRAGON EXERCISE

For the ancient Chinese, the dragon was a mythical creature which symbolized the Yang force of the Creative, the dynamic, electrically charged energy manifested in the thunderstorm. The flying dragon was always portrayed as being accompanied by rain, winds, clouds, and light-

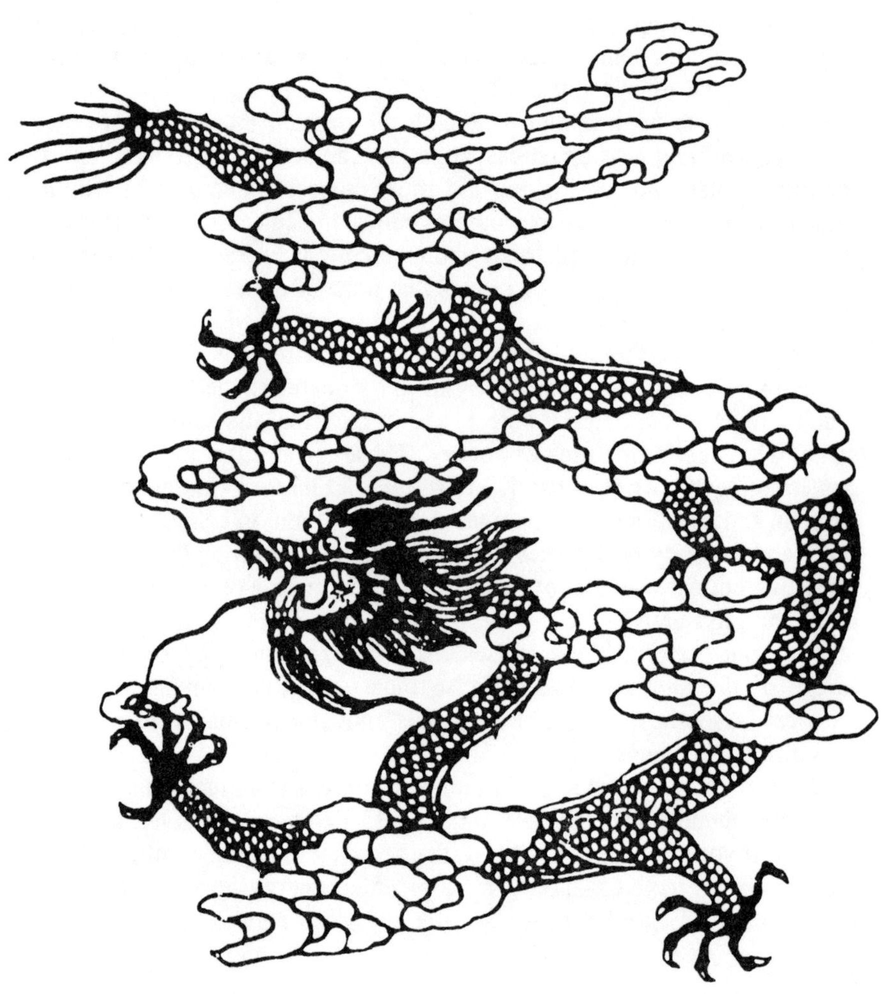

Illustration 3. The Dragon.

ning. The use of its image was reserved for personal use by the emperor, the Son of Heaven, as the dragon represented supreme wisdom, power, control, and social effectiveness.

The purpose of the Dragon Exercise is to instill the characteristics of the dragon into the mind and body of the practitioner. This exercise affects the mind by helping to overcome feelings of depression, anger, hostility, and all the anxieties brought on by being overwhelmed by adverse circumstances, for the dragon, flying through the heavens, is above all mundane concerns.

In some ancient Taoist texts, the Dragon Exercise appeared under other names. This was a precautionary measure taken to avoid political upheavals. The emperors have forbidden the common people from picturing themselves as dragons, because they would immediately rise up and dislodge the prevailing power.

Since the dragon represents the fire element, the physical effect of its exercise is to bring equilibrium to the heart, blood vessels, and absorption in the small intestines.

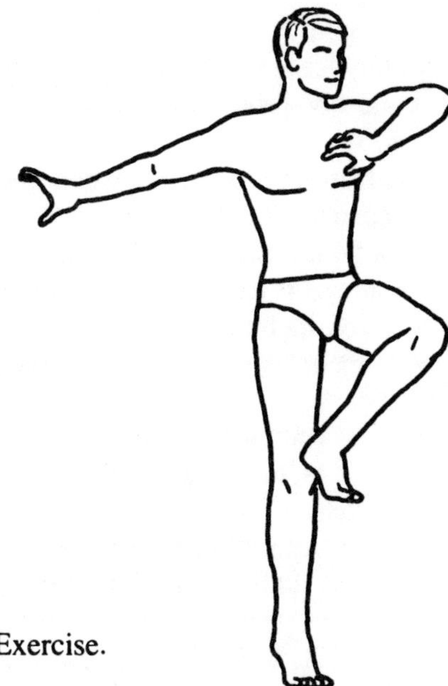

Figure 5. Dragon Exercise.

Begin the exercise by standing still. Then, take a few deep breaths while imagining as vividly as possible that you are a dragon with glowing eyes, open mouth with fangs, glistening emerald scales, curling tail, paws splayed showing long claws. Then, raising one foot, assume the pose and character of a dragon. While imagining that your hands are claws, hold one arm up with claws down and hold the other arm down with claws up. As this is not a formalized pose, a certain degree of freedom of expression is allowed within the confines of the image. Hold the pose as long as you can hold the image without straining. Repeat as many times as you comfortably can.

The most important aspect of this and all the other exercises is the union of the body and the mind. If the image fades or the mind wanders during the pose, stop and begin again. No benefit will be obtained unless the body and the mind are in union.

THE TIGER EXERCISE

While the dragon symbolizes the emperor, the tiger represents the general, a military leader with ambition, knowledge, power, and physical effectiveness and who protects the imperial throne and enforces the wishes of the emperor.

The tiger corresponds to the the wood element, so the Tiger Exercise affects the liver and nerves. The Taoists believe the structure of the nervous system is like a potted plant which sprouts from the liver.

The Tiger Exercise is useful in overcoming the adverse mental states of anxiety or hostility, ineffectualness, and lack of ambition. These adverse mental attitudes are believed to result from metabolic imbalances caused by liver dysfunction.

This exercise is recommended for healing and detoxifying the liver, to sooth inflamed nerves, to balance gallbladder functions, and to detoxify the brain and body cells.

The tiger demonstrates its power in its ability to capture something by leaping over it and grabbing it. The tiger pose is an imitation of this "leaping over" movement.

Begin by standing still. Take a few deep breaths while imagining yourself as a tiger. When the visualization is complete, bend your knees

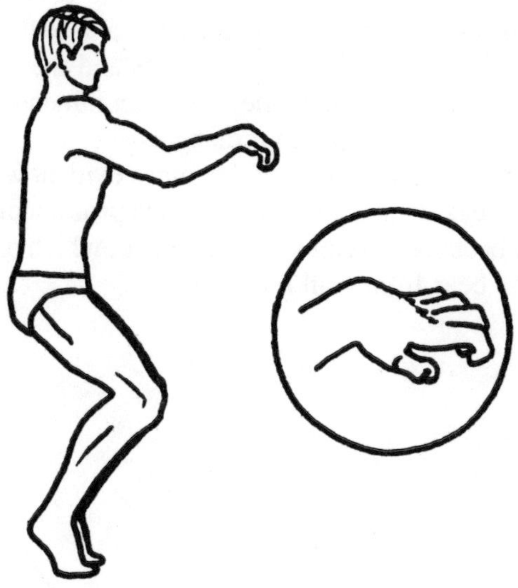

Figure 6. Tiger Exercise.

slightly and rise up on your toes while reaching up and out until your arms are straight. Keep the claws down, as if you have reached over and out to grab something. Maintain this position as long as you can hold the image without straining the body. Repeat as many times as is comfortable.

THE BEAR EXERCISE

The bear is also a very powerful animal, but it is an animal of leisure as well. Bears eat well, sleep well, wander about slowly, and are rather lazy and unaggressive. Bears are left alone and are not teased because they have the strength, courage, and prowess to deal with any potential adversary. The bear represents those who have attained a high degree of physical and material comfort. They can be successful business executives sitting behind large desks.

The Bear Exercise is recommended to aid the thought processes, to aid conceptualization, and to instill decisiveness into decision making.

The bear is associated with the earth element, and so this exercise affects the enzyme production of the spleen-pancreas and the functioning of the stomach muscle. This exercise is therefore recommended for bad digestion, hyper- and hypoglycemia, and diabetes.

The power and strength of the bear becomes evident when it stands and walks on its hind legs. In this position, the most prominent physical feature of the bear also becomes obvious—its stomach, which protrudes outward and prevents the bear from walking straight.

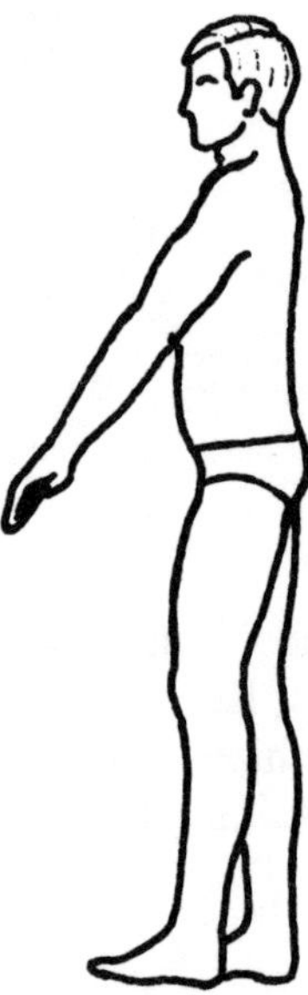

Figure 7. Bear Exercise.

Begin this exercise by standing still. Take a few deep breaths while visualizing yourself as a bear. Then with legs stiff, stomach pushed out, arms sloping out in front, walk slowly forward. As you do this, you will feel the movement of your abdomen and the stimulation of the area of the spleen-pancreas.

Continue walking this way as long as the image remains fixed in your mind. Repeat as many times as is convenient.

THE EAGLE EXERCISE

To the ancient Taoists the flying eagle represented the spirit because of its god-like qualities–silence, serenity, and invisibility. The eagle is also an accomplished hunter. It soars effortlessly to great heights, and its sharp eyes are alert to all details of the landscape below. The eagle manifests its attributes of intelligence, alertness, and ease when it hunts.

The eagle is associated with the metal element, so the Eagle Exercise stimulates the lungs, skin, and the large intestine.

This exercise is useful in overcoming melancholy, forlornness, and depression, which can result from or cause lung problems. (It is no coincidence that so many of the romantic poets and writers of Western literature suffered from tuberculosis.) This exercise is recommended for the treatment of emphysema, asthma, as well as skin problems (Taoists consider the skin to be the "third lung").

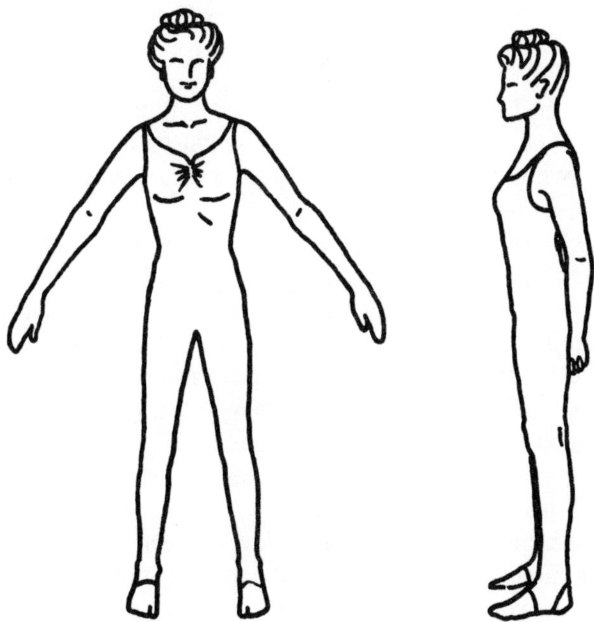

Figure 8. Eagle Exercise.

Outstretched wings effortlessly holding the eagle aloft mark the eagle. The reader should also remember that, when it is flying, the eagle's eyes are open and see everything.

Begin the Eagle Exercise by standing still. Take a few deep breaths while imagining yourself an eagle.

When the visualization is complete, begin to walk slowly with your arms held out to the side in a slant, or with your hands gently clasped behind you. As you walk, imagine you are an eagle, effortlessly floating through the blue sky, untouchable, divine. Your body should be very relaxed, but your mind and eyes should be very alert, noticing everything without focusing on any one thing in particular.

Continue the exercise as long as the mind does not wander. If it does, stop and begin again. Though this exercise can be performed anytime, anywhere, it is especially effective if done outdoors, after the evening meal.

THE MONKEY EXERCISE

To the ancient Taoists the monkey (or ape) epitomized boundless activity, curiosity, and free will. The monkey is constantly active, whether on the ground, swinging in the trees, or leaping playfully about, uninhibited by any cultural conventions.

The monkey is associated with the water element, so the Monkey Exercise stimulates the functions of the kidneys and bladder. This exercise is recommended for those feeling confined or restricted by circumstances in which there is a lack of freedom. To the Taoist will power resides in the kidneys. The Monkey Exercise is also recommended for any problems involving the kidneys, bladder, and urinary tract.

As the embodiment of free will, the monkey inspires an exercise that is free-style in the broadest sense. This exercise is best done in private as the presence of others might be inhibiting.

Begin by standing or sitting. Take a few deep breaths while imagining yourself as a monkey. When the visualization is complete, kick off your shoes, throw off your clothes, and begin to act like a little monkey. Sit on the floor, crouch in a chair, leap about, bounce up and down, hang upside down or by one arm, whatever is physically possible to do without strain or exertion.

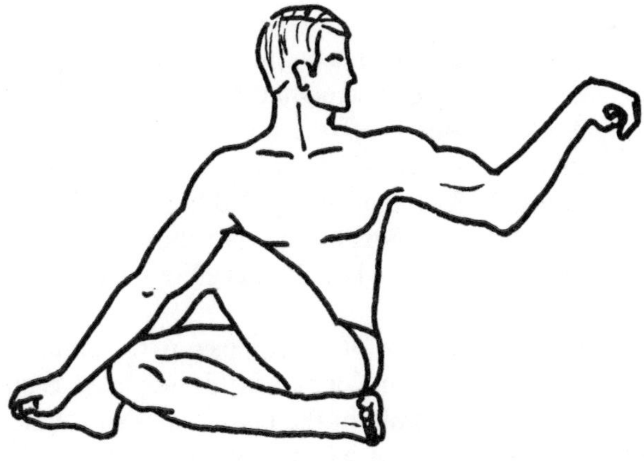

Figure 9. Monkey Exercise.

This exercise is completely free-style; all the movements and actions should act out impulses and whims as they occur to you. Monkeys also rub and scratch themselves a great deal. You may do this also, especially in the area of the kidneys.

EIGHT DIRECTIONAL EXERCISES

All the elements of the universe occupy space and are therefore directional. Since we are a part of the universe, we are influenced by space and are therefore directional also. Directionality arises wherever electric forces are present, and electric forces are everywhere because they are a property of atoms. The electric forces are the means whereby two magnets, for example, are drawn together or repelled apart. These forces are also the means whereby a weak magnet is made more powerful. This "recharging" of electrical forces involves correct orientation of a body, or "rechargee", with respect to the "recharger". For example, the north pole of a magnet must be placed against the south pole of another magnet in order for magnetic induction to take place. In magnets, as in other substances, "recharging" is actually a re-ordering of atoms or groups of atoms so that electrical energies are heightened.

It was after repeated experiments on the energizing properties of directionality that the Taoists developed eight directional exercises for energizing mankind. The exercises involve the execution of correct actions in correct directions. The forms of these exercises were modeled after the eight trigrams of the *Pa-Kua* and were called Eight Brocade Pieces. (The word "brocade" was used to express its preciousness to generations of people.) These exercises can also be called The Eight Directional Exercises or Eight Energizing Exercises.

Before you do these exercises, use a compass to determine the northern direction of the magnetic pole in your area (it is indicated as north by your compass), not the northern Pole of the earth's axis of rotation. Use this direction as a point of reference when doing the exercises.

The exercises are as follows:

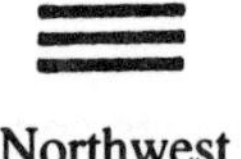

Northwest

For the Northwestern Exercise, orient the front of the body toward the northwest. Stand with the feet shoulder-width apart. Point the toes inward. This takes the pressure off the nerve endings in your heels and prevents imbalance in pressure. Now pretend you are lifting a barbell of medium weight (to prevent too much straining). While keeping

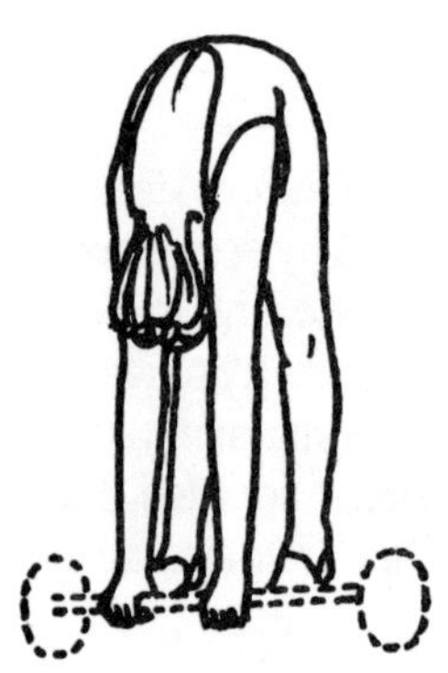

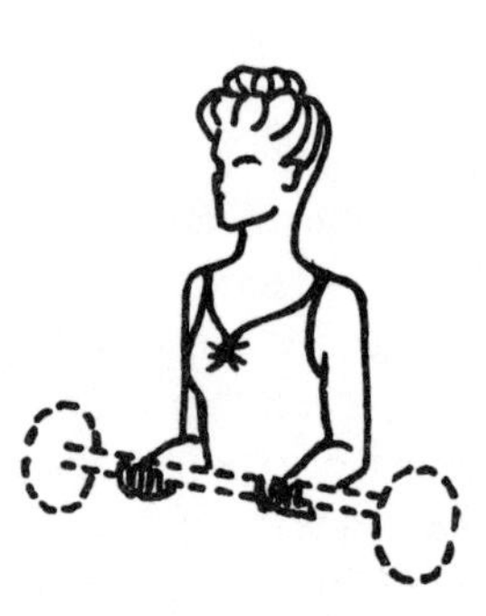

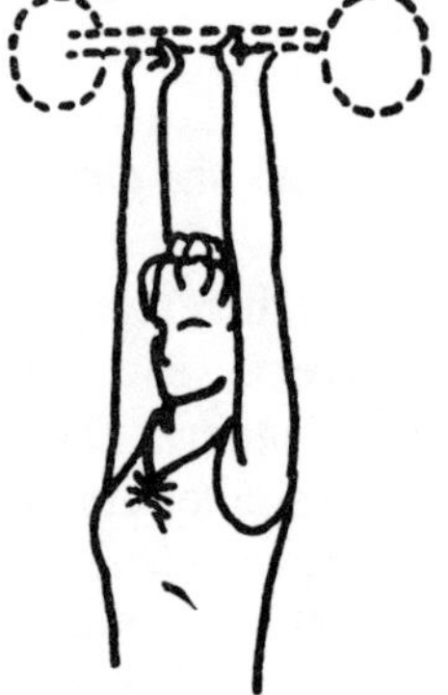

Figure 10. Northwestern Exercise.

the legs straight, bend down to pick up an imaginary barbell. Lift the barbell to waist level. Then lift the barbell as high as possible above your head. Really visualize that you are lifting a barbell. Then reverse this procedure. Do the exercise as many times as you wish. This exercise helps increase strength and benefits the lungs and large intestine.

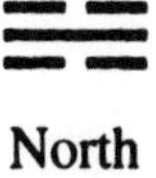

North

For the Northern Exercise, have your torso oriented in the northerly direction. Spread the feet wide apart. Pretend you are shooting an arrow from a bow. Shoot to your right and shoot to your left. Your head, arms, and torso change positions, but your feet remain stationary. Really visualize that you are pulling a taut bowstring and shooting an arrow. Do this exercise as many times as you wish. This exercise is good for the lungs, kidneys, large intestine, bladder, skin, and bones.

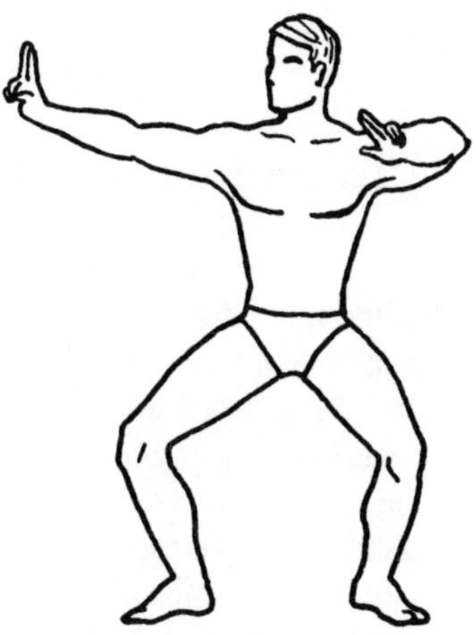

Figure 11. Northern Exercise.

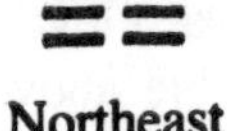

Northeast

Facing northeast, bend down and touch the toes with your fingertips. Keep the legs straight and bend at the waist and pelvis as much as possible. Then imagine that you are a mountain. This position may be held for as long as you wish. This exercise is good for the spleen-pancreas, muscle, and digestion.

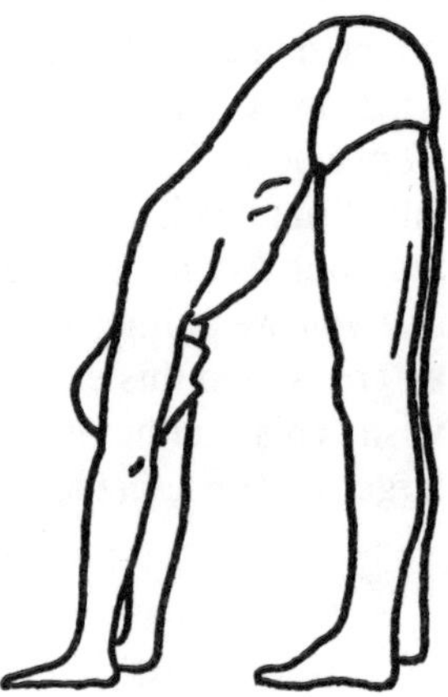

Figure 12. Northeastern Exercise.

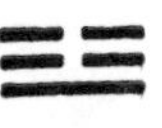

East

In the morning, stand under the sunlight and face east. Place your feet shoulder-width apart. Point the toes inward and close your eyes. With your arms hanging at your sides, turn the *upper body* to the right and left sides. Let your head turn with the torso, and let the eyeballs trace the source of radiant heat emitted by the sun. Never move your feet. Your mind should follow these movements—never let it wander. Do this as long as you like. This exercise is good for the nerves, liver, eyes, gallbladder, and weight reduction.

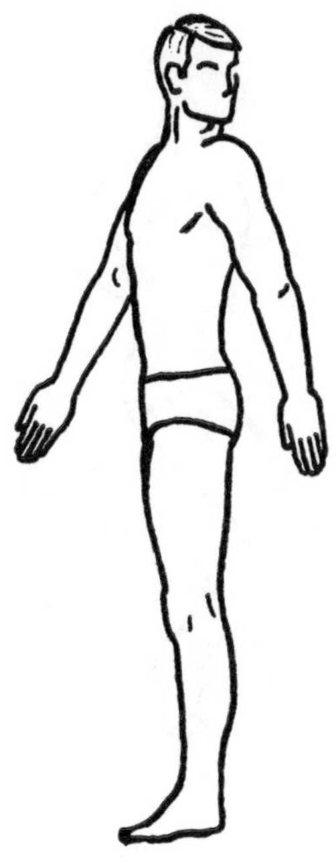

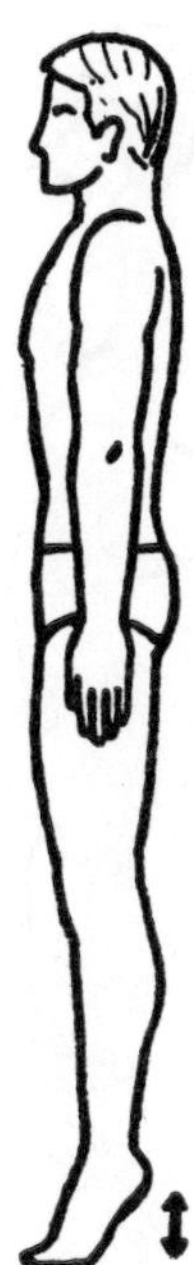

Figure 13. Eastern Exercise.

Figure 14. Southeastern Exercise.

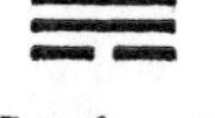

Southeast

Facing southeast, stand with your feet shoulder-width apart. Point your toes inward and raise yourself on your toes. Lower yourself. Do this seven times as a set. If you wish you may do more sets. Do not let your mind wander from your actions. This exercise benefits the nerves, liver, gallbladder, and heart.

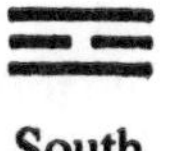

South

Facing south, rotate your hips as if you had a hoola-hoop around you. You may change the direction of rotation. Never let your mind wander onto other subjects. Do this as long as you wish. This exercise is good for the sexual organs.

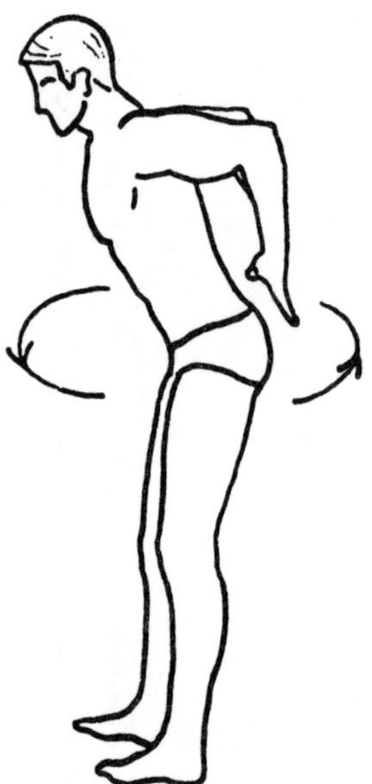

Figure 15. Southern Exercise.

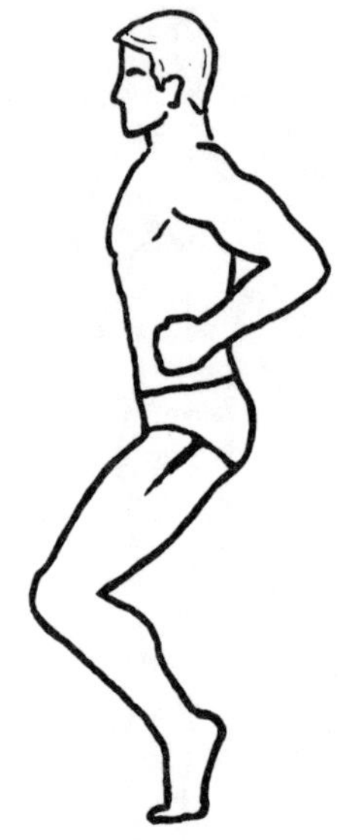

Figure 16. Southwestern Exercise.

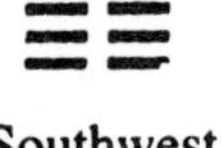

Southwest

Facing southwest, pose as if you were about to fight. Bend the knees slightly. Bend the arms slightly and clench the fists. Make your eyes bulge out with rage. Your mind must be with your body. Hold this pose as long as you wish. This exercise benefits the digestive system, lungs, and nerves.

West

Facing west, stand with your feet shoulder-width apart. Point the toes slightly inward. Raise one hand up in the air. Then bring the hand down and raise the other hand. Try to keep your abdomen still. As you do this your mind should follow these actions. Do this exercise as many times as you like, as this exercise helps lower back pain, shoulder pain, kidney problems, and spinal problems.

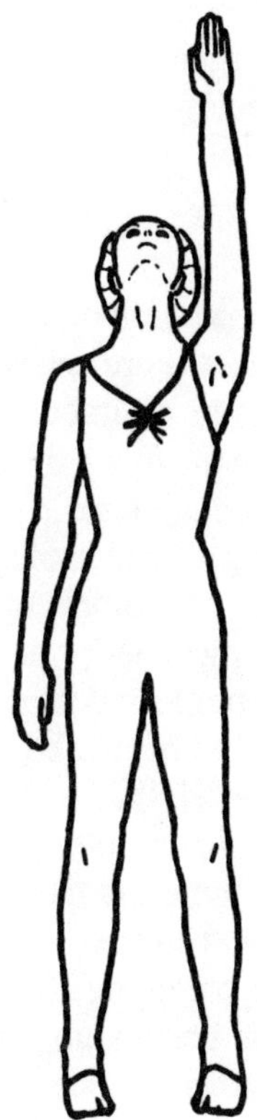

Figure 17.
Western Exercise.

These exercises are extremely versatile as they can be done anywhere, anytime. In two minutes, a homemaker, an executive, soldier, athlete, or anyone else can energize their tired bodies and minds. When the body is energized, business problems are solved easily, durability of the body is increased—anything is simplified.

TWELVE ZODIAC EXERCISES

Life is to live, and living is a function. This function is described by a Taoist formula, which is as follows:

Let f = function
o = organ
e = energy

$$f = o + e$$

In order to function, both organ and energy must be present. An organ without energy is dead. Pure energy without an organ is a ghost. Life will be meaningful—have a function—only when organ and energy are together. Apart from the many methods of harnessing and utilizing energy to balance the organ systems, Taoists have also created methods for maintaining the energy balance of specific organs. These involve the usage of time as measured by the biorhythmic clock to adjust imbalances by either dispersing (weakening) energy or toning (strengthening) energy.

Biorhythm—often referred to as the biological clock—is the regulation of the flow of energy within the body in relation to both solar and lunar time measurement. The word "biorhythm" encompasses all those concepts that denote the natural, inherent pulse underlying all functional aspects of life. In many ways this rhythm is taken for granted because being aware of it would, in a sense, be the same as being constantly aware of the rhythmical basis of one's own breathing. Because it has such a subtle and elusive nature, biorhythm is best exemplified when it is disrupted.

Jet fatigue—the consequence of suddenly traveling from one time zone to another—is a perfect example of how the body's natural rhythm is disrupted as a result of long-distance travel in a short period of time. It is sometimes difficult to conceive of the body functioning on a strict time schedule until one is abruptly placed in an environment regulated by a *different* schedule. The stress of having to readjust to an environment in relation to time makes one intensely aware of how rigidly scheduled the bodily functions are.

Taoists, after observing the circulation of energy throughout the body, formulated biorhythm cycles that precisely account for the energy flow along the meridian circuit during every second of the day. It was discovered that each of the main meridians has two-hour periods, called "watches", during which energy has a maximum intensity of circulation. For example, between 9 and 11 a.m., energy is at its peak in the spleen-pancreas meridian. It is during this time interval that the spleen-pancreas works the hardest. Between 11 a.m. and 1 p.m., when the energy activates the heart meridian, it is simultaneously at a minimum intensity in the spleen-pancreas meridian. There are twelve "watches" in a day, and they correspond to the twelve houses of the Zodiac. The following table lists the "watches" and the hours during which energy reaches its peak in each of the organs and bowels and their respective meridians.

Table 3. Biorhythm Cycles.

1–3 A.M.	Liver
3–5 A.M.	Lung
5–7 A.M.	Large Intestine
7–9 A.M.	Stomach
9–11 A.M.	Spleen-Pancreas
11–1 P.M.	Heart
1–3 P.M.	Small Intestine
3–5 P.M.	Bladder
5–7 P.M.	Kidney
7–9 P.M.	Heart Constrictor
9–11 P.M.	Triple Heater
11–1 A.M.	Gallbladder

Utilizing the biorhythm table will prove to be especially beneficial in pinpointing the specific organic causes of discomfort and balancing the energy level of that organ through the application of exercises that will either disperse or intromit energy, according to the needs of the organ. For example, if insomnia causes you to wake up between 1 and 3 o'clock in the morning regularly, a look at the table will tell you that the cause of the insomnia is a disorderly liver or nervous system. The aftereffects of insomnia—poor performance at work, tiredness, feeling of guilt, etc.—can be eliminated by applying the exercise appropriated for the 1 to 3 o'clock time interval. If you are constipated, the cause can be traced to untimely bowel movements. The recommended and biorhythmically determined time for bowel movements is from 5 to 7 o'clock in the morning. If you follow this schedule for bowel movements, you will not have to suffer from drugs, enemas, etc.

The exercises for these and other problems are called Twelve Zodiac Exercises, and they are listed in the order of the "watches" they correspond to. They are:

Watch A (1-3 a.m.) If ever you are awake during this time interval, you might want to sit with your legs crossed and try to see the tip of your nose. Drop your eyelids halfway to do this. Repeated attempts will enable you to see the tip of your nose. Also wrap the fingers around the thumb to make a closed fist and rest the fists on your knees. (Closing the fist retains the energy emitted from the fingers.) Breathe deeply and relax. Do this exercise for 5 to 30 minutes—the length of time is determined by you.

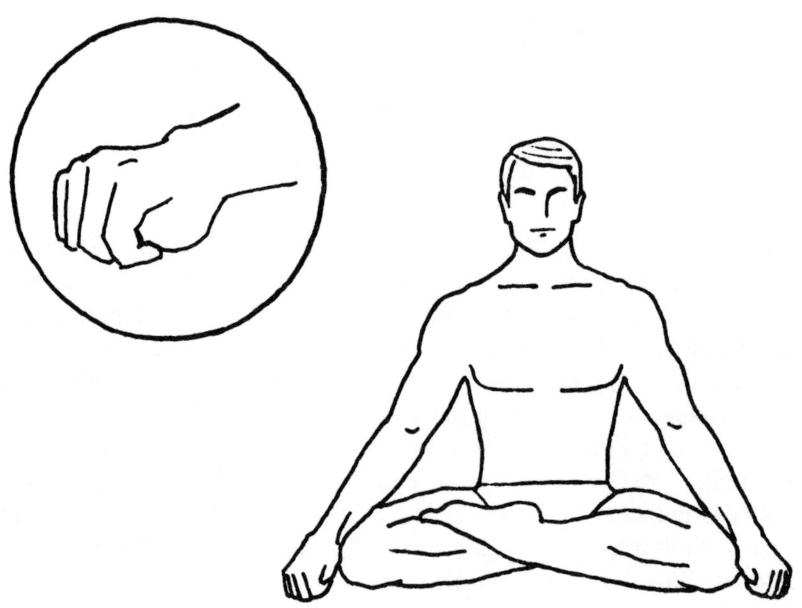

Figure 18. Watch A.

Watch B (3-5 a.m.) If ever you are awake during this time interval, sit with your legs crossed or in a position most comfortable to you. Close your eyes halfway and look at your nose. Do this as you hold your head by lacing your fingers behind the head and supporting with your palms. Then click your teeth. Deeply and slowly inhale and exhale nine times. Repeat this exercise for 5 to 30 minutes.

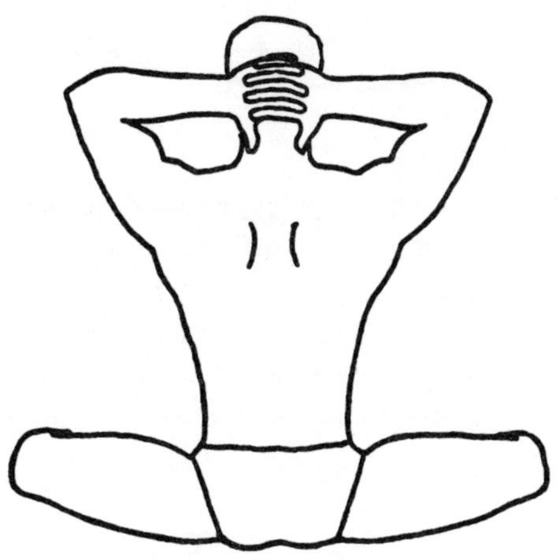

Figure 19. Watch B.

Watch C (5-7 a.m.) Cover the ears with the palms of your hands. Tap on the back of your head with your middle or index fingers so that a drum-like sound is made. This is called "Beating the Heavenly Drum". Then count your breaths. Inhale and count "one". Exhale and count "two". Inhale and count "three". And so on. Do this very slowly until you have reached the count of nine. (More about this exercise later.)

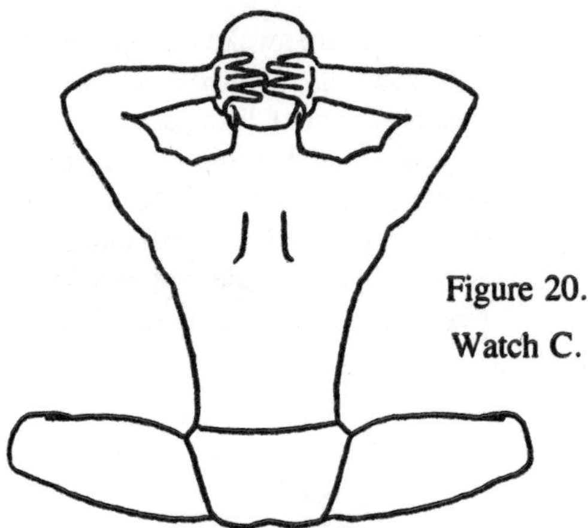

Figure 20.
Watch C.

Watch D (7-9 a.m.) Sit with your legs crossed. Now use your hands to hold the shins of your legs to support your upper body as you move your upper body around in circles. Make the circles as large as you can. Move freely. Reverse directions now and then to prevent dizziness. Do this exercise several times.

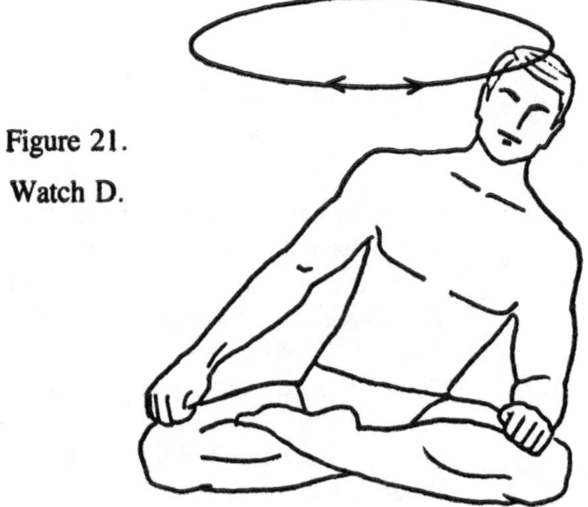

Figure 21.
Watch D.

Watch E (9-11 a.m.) Brush your teeth with your tongue. This creates saliva. Save the saliva until you have a mouthful. Then rinse your mouth with the saliva by swishing the saliva around in the your mouth as if it were mouthwash. Swallow the saliva slowly by dividing the mouthful of saliva into three swallows. Do this exercise several times. (More about this later.)

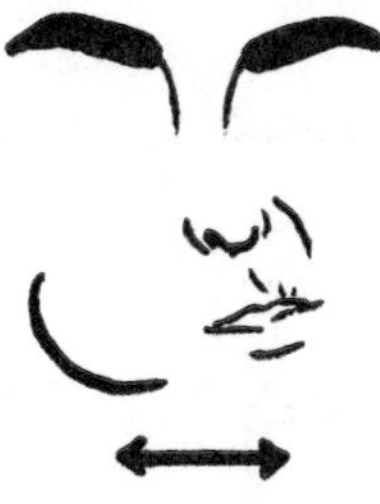

Figure 22.
Watch E.

Watch F
(11 a.m. to 1 p.m.) Remove clothing. Sit in a comfortable position. Inhale and hold your breath. Rub your hands together vigorously to generate heat and immediately place them on your back in the area of

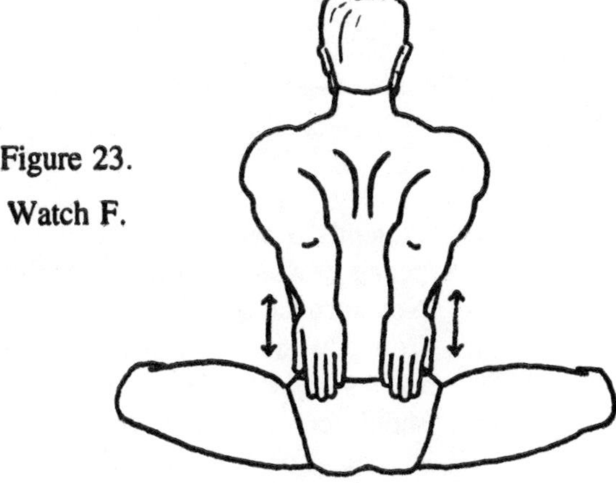

Figure 23.
Watch F.

the kidneys and rub until you cannot hold your breath any longer. Breathe and relax. Repeat the exercise.

Watch G (1-3 p.m.) For this exercise, sit comfortably. Inhale as deeply as you can. Feel the air come into your solar plexus, or the abdominal area. Use the navel as a center of focus. Then hold your breath to keep the air inside. Then try to feel a fire burning in the area. Concentrating on the fire will enable you to feel heat. Then exhale. This exercise is difficult to do, but repeated attempts will enable you to do it well.

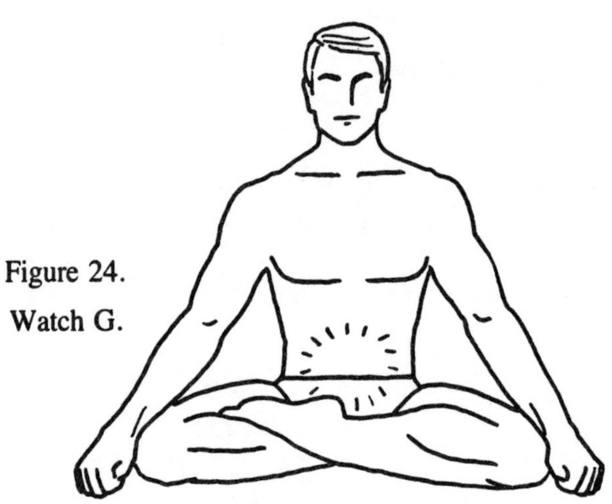

Figure 24.
Watch G.

Watch H (3-5 p.m.) Pretend that within each hand you are grasping the pedals of a bicycle (the hands should form a fist). Now turn the pedals so that one hand moves away from you on the down-stroke while the other hand moves toward you on the up-stroke. Each hand should complete eighteen turns. This completes one set. You can repeat the exercise if you wish.

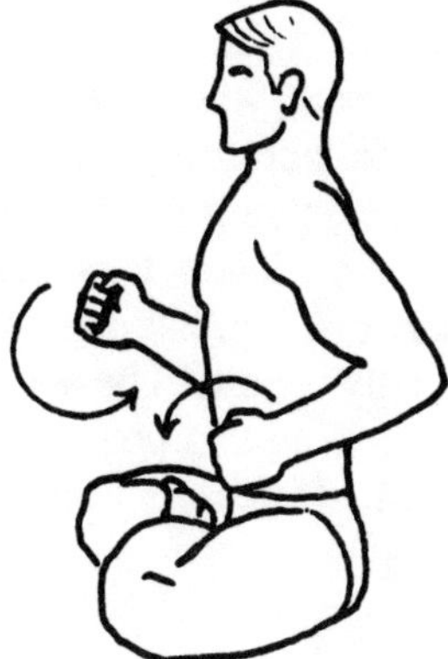

Figure 25.
Watch H.

Watch I (5-7 p.m.) Sit on the floor or the bed with your legs outstretched flat. Then lace your fingers and—palms up—reach for the ceiling, as far as you can go. Feel your back and side muscles stretch. When you are tired, rest your hands on your head. Then lift them up again. Breathe normally. The exercises may be repeated as many times as you wish.

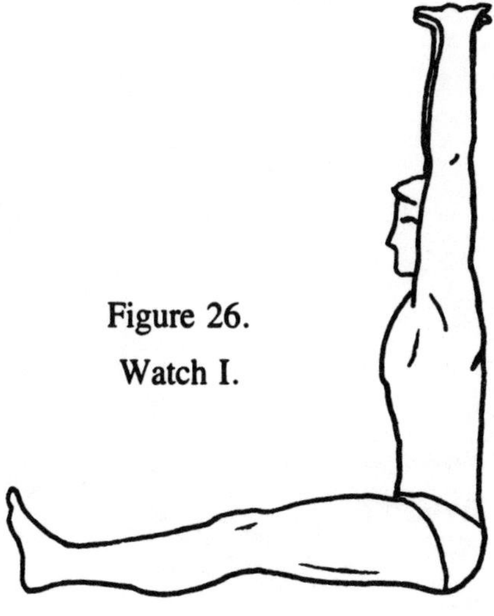

Figure 26.
Watch I.

Watch J (7-9 p.m.) Sit on the floor with your legs outstretched. Reach forward and try to touch your toes. Then try to touch the soles of your feet. If you cannot reach your toes, do not force yourself. Then relax. Again assume the initial sitting position. Now pat your upper legs, lower legs, and thighs. Relax. Then repeat the exercise as many times as you can. Gradually, you will be able to grab the soles of your feet. Hold this position until you can no longer hold it. Release and relax.

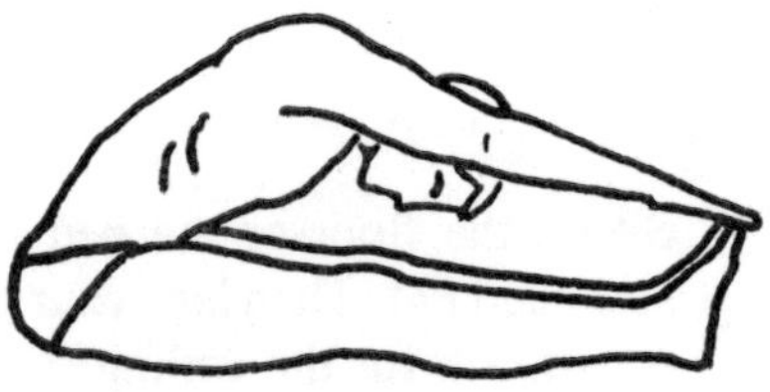

Figure 27. Watch J.

Watch K (9-11 p.m.) Follow the procedures for Watch E.

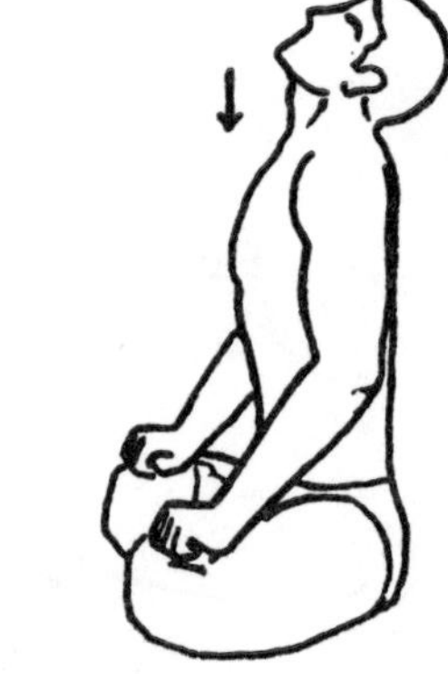

Figure 28. Watch K.

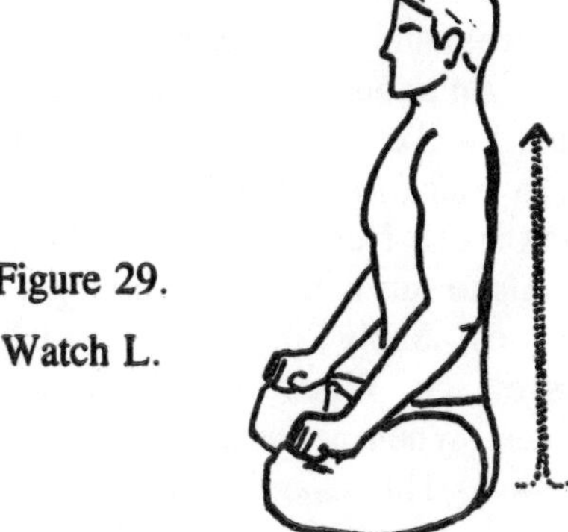

Figure 29.
Watch L.

Watch L (11 p.m. to 1 a.m.) Follow the procedures for Watch G, but as you hold your breath, tighten the muscles of your rectum as much as possible and as long as possible. Try to feel a tingling sensation shoot up your spine. Release, relax, and exhale slowly. Repeat this exercise several times. This is also a difficult exercise that can be mastered after continuous practice.

TWELVE NERVE EXERCISES

2,000 years ago during the Han Dynasty, a man from the West went to China and devoted his entire life to the study and practice of Taoism and a form of Buddhism. His name was Dharma and he lived in the White Horse Temple in the capital of the Han Empire.

His book, *The Text of Altering Nerves*, was the result of his lifework. It contained only a few pages of complex verses which obscured vital information for increasing the practitioner's longevity. (In those days, such information was hidden from those who would make light of it.)

In his book Dharma stated that all human problems were caused by problems within the nervous system and that human beings could live longer if they "altered" (renewed) their nervous system. In so doing, Dharma furthered mankind's comprehension of the nervous system.

The nerves are an intricate and elaborate network of "communication cables" connecting our brain to our organs and our organs to our organs. One break in your "cable" will cause your body to suffer. For example, if tension chokes a nerve in your finger, your finger will soon atrophy, and you will be forced to cut it off. Nerve cells need chemicals produced by interaction with other cells to survive, and the functions of other cells are dependent upon the nerves. Sadly, our nerves shrink and harden after we reach twenty years of age. When nerves deteriorate, impulses are conducted at slower rates. When nerve impulses are slow, mental and physical processes are slow. This is aging. Young people below twenty years of age have nerves that are soft and expandable.

To remain youthful, we must exercise our nerves to reverse deterioration and to preserve softness and expansibility. Dharma developed twelve exercises, called Twelve Nerve Exercises, which soften and expand our nervous system. Their movements recall those of T'ai Chi Chuan, although the theoretical basis of the nerve exercises differ from those of T'ai Chi Chuan. Although T'ai Chi Chuan may have stemmed from the nerve exercises (it was developed by Taoist master Chang San-Fung 1700 years later than the nerve exercises), it is used for combat purposes, whereas the Twelve Nerve Exercises are used for removing stress and tension and preserving the nervous system.

The Twelve Nerve Exercises unite the mind and body in order to bring about relaxation. If you have ever tried to relax your entire body with your mind—a concept employed by biofeedback machines—you will find that relaxation of the body is difficult to achieve. Relaxing the body with the mind involves clearing your mind of all thoughts. This in itself is a difficult feat because your mind is always cluttered with thoughts. Dharma, acknowledging the fact that the mind is always active, made the mind follow series of body movements that would lead both mind and body to a state of relaxation, as relaxation is the first step to preservation. If we can preserve our nervous system by renewing a deteriorating nervous system, we can live longer and preserve our youth.

Each exercise leads to the next; therefore, all twelve exercises must be done in their proper order. The exercises, in their original order, are as follows:

1. Stand with your feet shoulder-width apart. Direct toes inward.

(Do not face south when doing the exercise.) Place palms on breasts so that the middle three fingers of each hand meet over the thymus gland. Feel the heart beat. Smile and imagine you are humble and polite. (This action relaxes the body by removing the spirit of contention.)

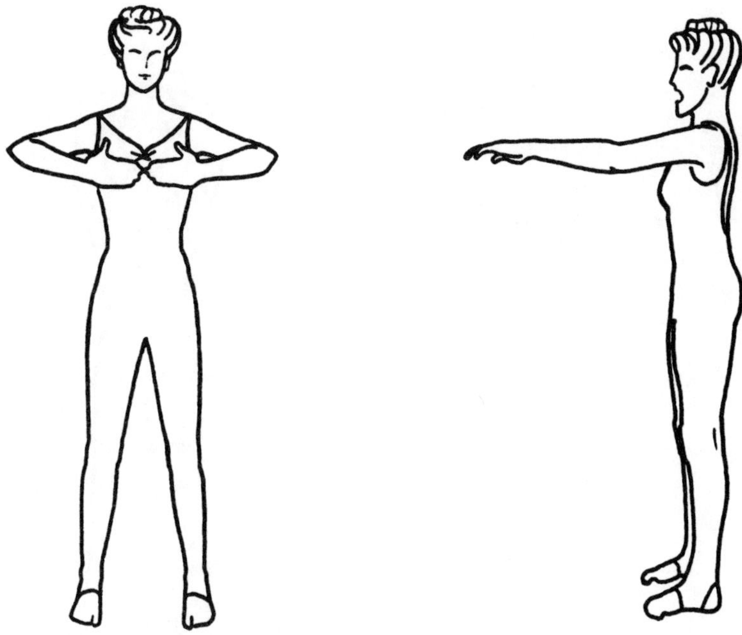

Figure 30. First Pose. Figure 31. Second Pose

2. While holding the first pose, spread your toes apart and dig them into the ground as if they were claws clutching at something. Open your mouth and look blankly ahead, as if you were a fool. (A fool does not seek knowledge or betterment and is therefore relaxed.) Then move the hands outward with palms down and fingers bent loosely. Hold them there.

3. Continuing from the previous pose, stand on your toes. Then clench your teeth. Then lace your fingers and lift them, palms up, as high as you can stretch. Then lower yourself until you are standing with your feet flat on the ground.

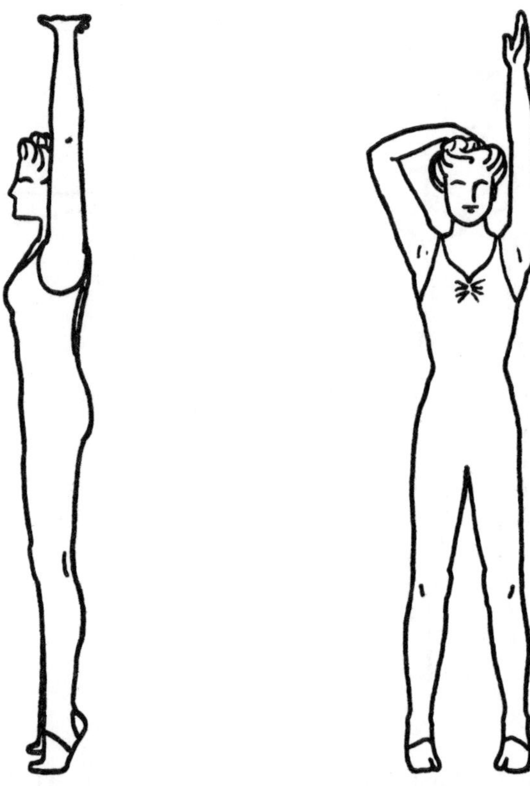

Figure 32. Third Pose.

Figure 33. Fourth Pose.

4. While holding the previous pose, put one hand on your head to prevent it from moving (keep the other hand up) while the eyes move forcefully from side to side. Now repeat this exercise using the other hand to prevent the head from moving.

5. If the hand held straight is the right hand, move the right leg forward; if the hand held straight is the left hand, move the left leg forward. The hand held straight moves down and makes an overhand fist. (All fists should be made with the thumb hidden inside the fingers.) The hand from on top of the head moves to the side and forms an underhand fist (while doing so, bend the elbow). Your eyes should be fixed on the overhand fist. Switch arm positions. Switch arm positions again and again. The movements made should be similar to karate arm movements.

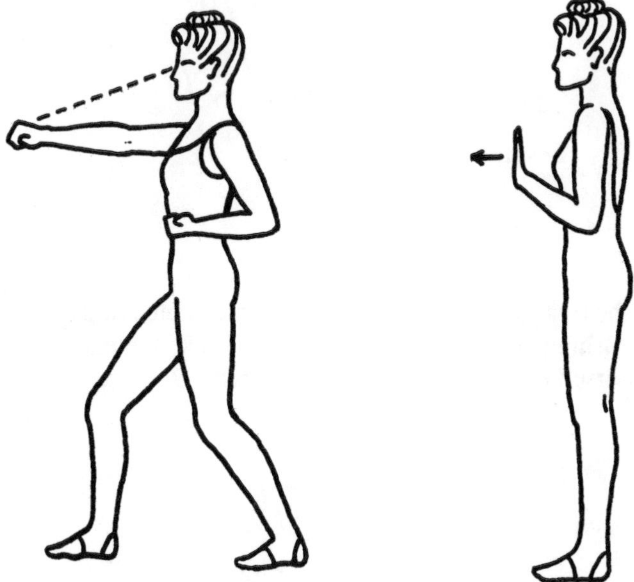

Figure 34. Fifth Pose. Figure 35. Sixth Pose.

6. Adopt the first pose, but make underhand fists at your side. Bulge out your eyes as if you were angry. Bring the fists up. Now they are in an overhand position. Push, but slowly as if you are pushing somebody. Your right eye should be fixed upon the right fist and the left eye should be fixed upon the left fist. Then quickly and forcefully pull the arms back so that fists are underhand again. Then repeat the exercise seven times. Then relax the entire body, including the eyes.

7. Put one hand under your chin and one hand over your head and turn your head to the right and left sides. Switch hand positions and turn the head again. Do this three or four times.

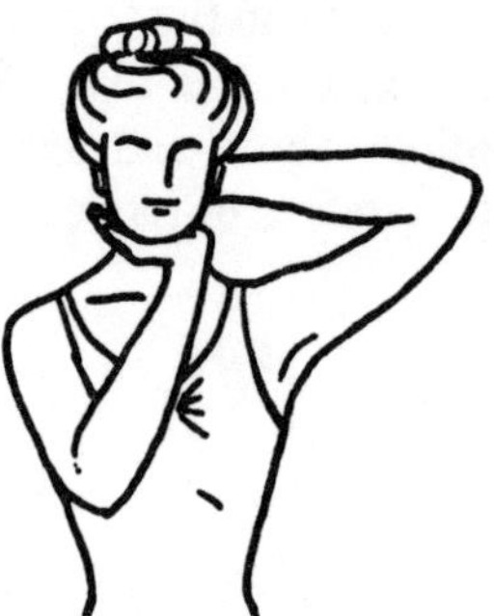

Figure 36.
Seventh Pose.

8. Adopt the first pose. Now stoop down, while pretending that your arms are pushing something down. As you sink, pretend you are pushing yourself down. Stand up and sink again. Do so seven times.

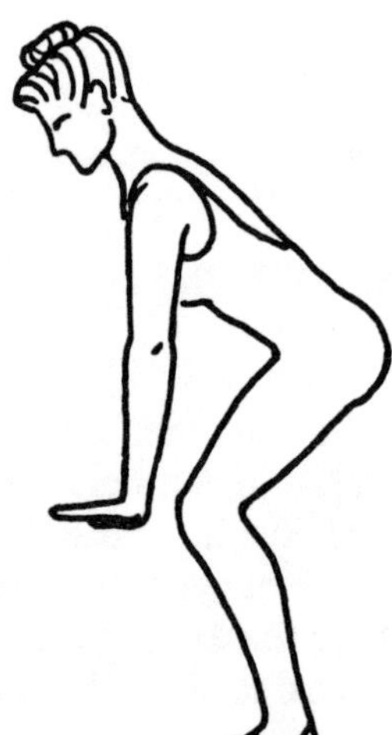

Figure 37.
Eighth Pose.

9. Adopt the first pose. Follow the instructions for exercise number five, only this time the fingers are rounded (no fists) and the arms are close together. Move the arms out and in and feel the effects on the arm and back muscles. Then relax. Repeat exercise.

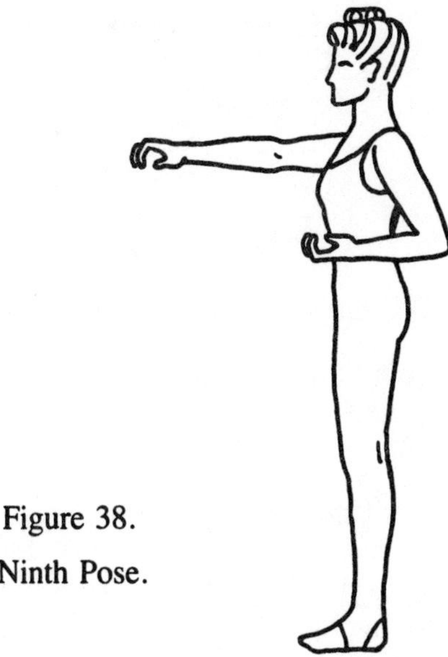

Figure 38.
Ninth Pose.

10. Begin with the first pose. Then relax and bend over and walk forward on your fingers until you are on your toes. If you cannot do this, walk on your hands. Hold this position until you can no longer hold it. Later, you may try walking on your middle three fingers.

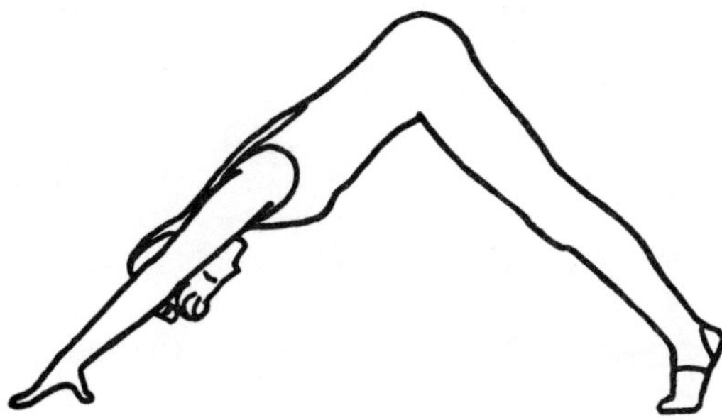

Figure 39. Tenth Pose.

11. Move to the first pose. Lace your fingers and place them behind your head and bend down. Close your eyes while doing this. Then raise your upper body to return to the original position.

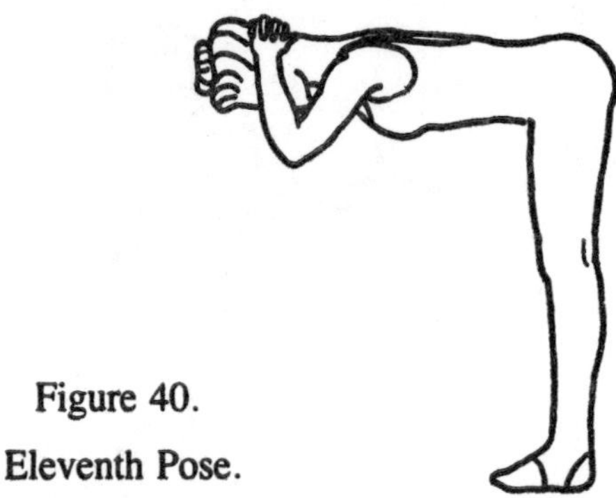

Figure 40.
Eleventh Pose.

12. Keep holding your hands behind your head and bend the upper body forward, pushing one leg back. Keep one leg forward and bent. Then use your bent leg to push the body into a standing position. Then sink down again, pushing the other leg back. Then return to center position and adopt the first pose. After you have placed your hands in the heart position, you will have finished the exercise series.

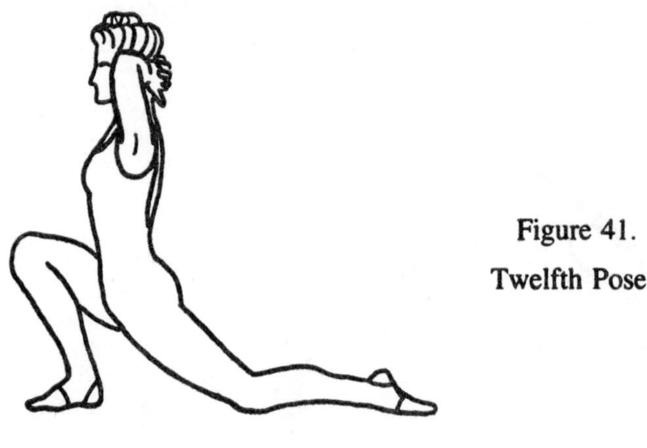

Figure 41.
Twelfth Pose.

THE DEER EXERCISE FOR MEN

The Five Animal Exercises, Eight Directional Exercises, Twelve Zodiac Exercises, and Twelve Nerve Exercises are for general healing. In addition to these, the Tao of Revitalization offers approximately a thousand other exercises that energize and strengthen individual parts or areas of the body and deal with specific health problems. In the following paragraphs most of these exercises will be dwelt with in full.

Thousands of years ago, Taoist sages selected three animals which were noted for longevity from the many: the deer, the crane, and the turtle. One of these, the deer, was also noted for its strong sexual and reproductive abilities. The sages minutely observed the behavior that seemed to contribute to the deer's abilities. They saw that the deer exercised its anus when it wiggled its tail. After studying the results of the exercise, the sages immediately adopted the principle and re-designed it for human use. Thus, the Deer Exercise was born.

The Deer Exercise achieves six important objectives. First of all, it builds up the tissues of the sexual organs. Secondly, it draws energy up through six of the seven glands of the body into the pineal gland to elevate spirituality. (There is a hormone pathway that leads from the prostate, connects with the adrenal glands, and continues on to the other glands.) Concurrently, blood circulation in the abdominal area is increased. This rush of blood helps transport the nutrients and "life force" (energy) of the semen to the rest of the body.

When energy is brought up into the pineal gland, a chill or tingling sensation is felt to ascend through the spine to reach the head. This sensation should feel somewhat like a climax. If you feel a sensation in the area of the pineal gland, but do not feel the tingling sensation in the middle of your back, do not worry. Your sensitivity will increase with experience. If after some time you still cannot sense the progress of energy, certain problems must be taken care of first.

Self-determination is the third benefit derived from the Deer Exercise. If one gland in the Seven Glands System is functioning below par, the energy shooting up the spine will stop there. This indicates a weakness, and special attention should be given to that area. For example, if the thymus gland is functioning poorly, the energy will stop there, and the energy will continue to stop there until the thymus gland is healed. When the thymus is again functioning normally, the energy will then move further up along the spine toward the pineal gland. If the energy moves all the way up to your head during the Deer Exercise, it indicates that all the seven glands are functioning well and that there is no energy blockage in the body. On the other hand, if you do not feel anything during the Deer Exercise, a blockage is indicated. The movement of energy can be felt by everyone if no dysfunctions are encountered.

The fourth benefit of the Deer Exercise is that it builds up sexual ability and enables the man to prolong sexual intercourse. During *ordinary* intercourse the prostate swells with semen to maximum size before ejaculating. During ejaculation, the prostate shoots out its contents in a series of contractions. Then, sexual intercourse ends. With nothing left to ejaculate, induce contractions, or maintain an erection (energy is lost during ejaculation), the man cannot continue to make love. But, if he uses the Deer Exercise to pump semen out of the prostate in small doses, pumping it in the other direction into the other glands and blood vessels, he can prolong intercourse.

Under ordinary circumstances, when the Deer Exercise is not used during intercourse, it will be harmful to interrupt orgasm or prolong intercourse by ordinary means. Under ordinary means, the prostate remains expanded for a long time, unrelieved by the pumping action of ejaculation, until the semen is carried away by the blood stream. But the prostate is somewhat like a rubber band: it must be allowed to snap back to its original form, otherwise continuous extension will bring about a loss of elasticity. When the prostate loses its elasticity, its function is impaired and it is damaged. The Deer Exercise prolongs orgasm and intercourse, but it protects the prostate by relieving it.

The fifth benefit to be derived from the exercise, needless to say, is that it builds up sexual energy. It does so by generating and balancing the secretions of the endocrine glands, particularly the sexual glands.

Often as a person experiences this increase in sexual energy, the tendency is to increase one's sexual exploits. Taoism allows for this possibility, but views promiscuity as a violation of the natural laws of healing. Anything, when carried to excess, leads to weakness or depletion of energy. On the other hand, leading a normal and active sexual life, while doing nothing to rebuild the lost energy which has been given up during sexual relations, is like burning a candle at both ends. One secret of continual youth is to maintain a reserve of energy by having strong sexual organs. This is one effect of the Deer Exercise. (There is also a special treatise on the proper handling of the consequent increased sexual energy with respect to sexual relationships and intercourse. As it would be impossible to go into a lengthy discourse here, *The Tao of Sexology* is recommended for further research.)

The sixth effect of the exercise is to strengthen the anal muscles and rectum. As one grows old and weak, one's anal opening tends to become very loose and flaccid. This is why many older persons, or those who have lost the use of the nerves which control the anus, through either paralysis or stroke, have a difficult time controlling their bowels. Anal muscles which have atrophied and become weak hasten the onset of diseases, such as hemorrhoids and prostate cancer. Thus one secret of maintaining youth into one's old age is to exercise these muscles and keep them strong.

In the male, the prostate lies behind the anal muscles. When the sphincter muscles are contracted, the prostate is exercised and strengthened. This helps prevent or even reverse many diseases associated with the prostate, such as enlargement through overuse or dysfunction through weakness and cancer. This is a boon to males over forty years of age who tend to suffer from problems of the prostate.

The Deer is therefore a physical exercise as well as a mental and spiritual one. It improves one's sexual abilities as it builds up the energy reserves within the body. Fertility is increased and strengthened. Over time, the mental processes are heightened as well, and the outcome is often an increase in psychic powers and the growing feeling of an inner tranquility, which is a necessary prerequisite for the unfolding of one's spiritual centers.

INSTRUCTIONS FOR THE MALE DEER EXERCISE

This exercise may be done standing, sitting, or lying down. Do this exercise in the morning upon rising and before retiring at night.

First Stage:

(The purpose of this stage is to encourage semen production.)

1. Rub the palms of your hands together vigorously. This creates heat in your hands by bringing the energy of your body into your

hands and palms.

2. With your right hand, cup your testicles so that the palm of your hand completely covers them. (This exercise is best done without clothing.) Do not squeeze. Just a slight pressure should be felt, as well as the heat from your hand.

3. Place the palm of your left hand on the area of your pubis, one inch below your navel.

4. With a slight pressure so that a gentle warmth begins to build in the area of your pubis, move your left hand in clockwise or counter-clockwise circles eighty-one times.

5. Rub your hands together vigorously again.

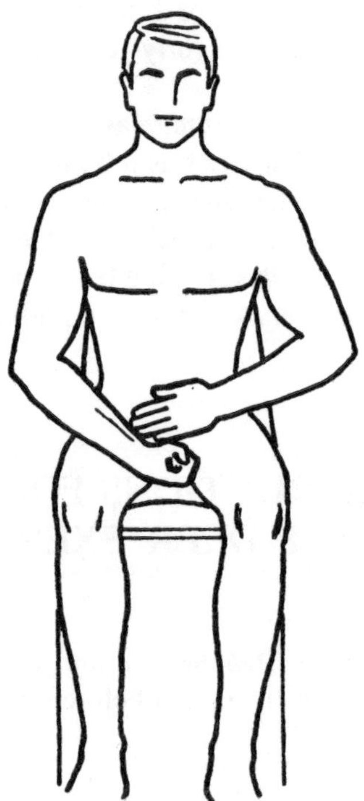

Figure 42. The Male Deer Exercise.

6. Reverse the position of your hands so that your left hand cups your testicles and your right hand is on your pubis. Repeat the circular rubbing in the opposite direction another eighty-one times. Concentrate on what you are doing, and feel the warmth grow. For all Taoist exercises, it is very important—even necessary—that you concentrate on the purpose of the physical motions, for doing so will enhance the results. It will unify the body and mind to bring full power to your purpose. Never try to use the mind to force the natural processes by imagining fires growing in the pubic area. The use of imagination does not apply to this exercise.

Second Stage:

1. Tighten the muscles around your anus and draw them up and in. When done properly it will feel as if air is being drawn up your rectum, or as if your entire anal area is being drawn in and upward. Tighten as hard as you can and hold as long as you are able to do so comfortably.

2. Stop and relax a moment.

3. Repeat the anal contractions. Do this as many times as you can without feeling discomfort. At first you may find that you are able to hold the anal sphincter muscles tight for only a few seconds. Do not be discouraged and please persist. After several weeks you will be able to hold the muscles tight for quite a while without experiencing weariness or strain.

NOTE A: As you do the second stage of the exercise, you should concentrate on feeling a tingling sensation (similar to an electric shock) ascend along the pathway of the seven glands. The sensation lasts for fractions of a second and results naturally. Do not try to force this with mental images.

Some teachings suggest that thoughts should be used to help or guide energy flow. Those who make these suggestions misunderstand the nature of energy.

There are six forms of energy: mechanical energy, heat energy, sound energy, radiant energy, atomic energy, and electrical energy. We emit electrical energy. The electrical energy in man differs drastically from that used to run a house. The electrical current in the average home fluctuates at 60 cycles per second; in men, 49,000,000 cycles per second. The latter figure is about half that of light, which travels at 186,000 miles per second. So when a man starts to think, breathe, or visualize to help the energy reach its destination, the electrical energy will have already reached its destination. Our thoughts, breaths, etc. are too slow to guide the flow of electrical energy.

What occurs at the unconscious level was not meant to be subject to the control of the conscious mind. If the conscious mind interferes with something it was not evolved to control—helping or guiding electrical energy through visualization, thoughts, etc.—it can cause a great deal of mental and physical damage. Its interference with the natural progress of energy can cause schizophrenia, brain damage, and other problems. Taoists call these calamities "Disintegration into Evil". I have personally seen many such disintegrations in the East and West.

The Deer Exercise is extremely safe—provided, that is, it is not supplemented with techniques of other teachings. For show, various incompatible techniques are often thrown together to create spectacular techniques, but the results are often disastrous. Lao-Tse said, "My way is simple and easy." And true Taoist methods *are* simple and easy.

NOTE B: To determine whether or not the Deer Exercise is having an effect on the prostate gland, try this test: as you urinate, try to stop the stream of urine entirely through anal muscle contractions. If you are able to do so, then the exercise is effective.

NOTE C: If an erection occurs while practicing this exercise, then place the thumb of the hand cupping the testicles at the base of the penis next to the pubis and press down sharply, while massaging the area of the pubis with the other hand. This will inhibit the flow of blood into the penis and maximize the build-up of energy within the sexual glands. (Tao of Sexology deals with the issue of proper orgasm without ejaculation to control the loss of energy during masturbation or sexual intercourse. The teachings stress that one does not wish to experience ejaculation following this exercise, or at other times, except for purposes of procreation, as this dissipates the energy which has begun to build as a consequence of this exercise. Taoism stresses the use of this energy for elevating spirituality, so that mankind can meet physical, mental, and spiritual aspirations at one time.)

NOTE D: Always concentrate on what you are doing.

Proper hygiene must be practiced in conjunction with the exercise. We need to take the time daily to wash our entire bodies, including all the openings to the body. Social mores train us to wash the face, mouth, and teeth thoroughly. But we often neglect to wash the anal opening due to social taboos surrounding this particular area of the body. Please, take the time to clean the anal opening and the genitals so that germs and feces do not have a chance to collect, which can lead to infections, cancers, hemorrhoids or other weaknesses in this area of the body. Refer also to the Sun Worship Exercise.

Pressure is being placed on the prostate gland as it is gently massaged by the tightening action of the anal muscles. (The anus can be thought of as a little motor which pumps the prostate gland.) Thus stimulated, the prostate begins to secrete hormones such as endorphins, which produce a natural high. When the prostate goes into spasms, a small orgasm is experienced. By alternately squeezing and relaxing the anus during the Deer Exercise, a natural high is produced without having to jog ten or more miles or endure its side-effects.

Among other things, this exercise cures and prevents hemorrhoids and cures problems of the prostate, such as weakness, enlargement, and cancer. It strengthens the nerve endings around the pubis and penis and may be used to correct problems of impotence and premature ejaculation. Contraction of the anal muscles will also help enlarge the head or bulb of the penis, which will give the man more pleasant sensations during sexual intercourse.

It is crucial to learn control over the anal muscles if one is to master the later meditative and breathing Internal Exercises. These muscles may be described as a door or a lock. When shut, they close off the upper body and allow the energy to collect and build in the abdominal channel. Without this build-up of energy, it will be impossible to properly stimulate the sexual organs, and in turn, the other glands of the body. It is essential then to gain mastery over this lock if one is to strengthen one's system sufficiently to begin to energize the spiritual centers in the body.

THE DEER EXERCISE FOR WOMEN

The benefits women can derive from the Deer Exercise are numerous and noteworthy.

Taoism provides a way for a woman to eliminate the problems related to the menstrual period, even in the middle of a period. These problems include emotional ups and downs, water retention, hormone blockages, cramps, and abnormal flow of blood. (A light menstrual flow indicates blockage and body poisoning. If the period suddenly stops—without the influence of the Deer Exercise—disease is indicated.)

The exercise strengthens the muscles of the rectum and prevents and/or cures hemorrhoids. It cures and prevents vaginal problems such as infections, discharges, colitis, and leucorrhea. It increases the circulation in the sexual organs and energizes the pubic area.

The vagina greatly benefits from the Deer Exercise. It becomes tighter, meatier, and more flexible. So a woman who has had children can greatly benefit from the Deer, as the man's pleasure is increased during intercourse. (Childbirth can leave the vagina loose and enlarged, resulting in a great loss of penile sensation for her partner during intercourse.) By performing the exercise, a woman can energize and tighten her vagina.

In addition, the Deer stimulates natural estrogen production. The exercise stimulates the production of the female hormone estrogen and causes it to spread throughout the vagina, uterus, breasts, and ovaries. A surge in estrogen levels can greatly relieve the symptoms of menopause and rejuvenate a woman. For thousands of years, the Deer was effectively used for maintaining a youthful countenance. Historical records show that women famous for their beauty consistently use the technique. An added benefit is that the increase in estrogen results naturally and that the body naturally balances the increased estrogen level with other substances.

The fact that estrogen is produced naturally is very important. The body knows what amount of estrogen it needs at any given time. A doctor administering man-made estrogen, a drug that is not balanced with the other substances normally occurring within the body, cannot know what exact level of the hormone is needed in the bloodstream. Every hour the hormone level in the blood changes and it would be impossible to follow it. Moreover, man-made estrogen will eventually cause problems by either over- or under-dosing. The body is the best judge of the amount of estrogen to be released, because its sensitive sensors are on the alert every second of the day.

Furthermore, the exercise provides a way for a young, fertile woman to eliminate her menstrual period in a safe way. If the Deer Exercise, parts one and two, is performed over a period of time, menstruation ceases and countless other benefits emerge.

Normally every month, the outer linings of the uterine walls thicken with blood vessels for the anticipated implantation of the fertilized egg. If an egg is fertilized by a sperm, it attaches to the thickened walls and begins to invade the nutrient-rich walls. Absorbing nutrients from the blood, the egg grows continuously until it becomes a fully-developed baby. If fertilization of the egg never occurs, no implantation will take place and the thick lining of blood will be sloughed off, because it is no longer needed. A great deal of blood and nutrients are lost during the monthly sloughings, or menstruation.

The Deer stops this monthly loss of blood. Some women are reluctant to stop menstruation because they think it is "unnatural". But there is no need to worry. Cessation of menstruation is actually not a strange event: menstruation stops immediately during menopause, pregnancy, or nursing.

When a woman is pregnant, the body instinctively absorbs the supply of blood and directs all of it to the thriving egg. The blood and energy normally lost during menstruation are then used by the sexual glands in particular to benefit the fetus. After birth, if the mother nurses the newborn, menstruation will not immediately resume, as the blood will be directed to the breasts for conversion to milk.

By stopping menstruation with the Deer Exercise, a phenomenon referred to as "Turning Back the Blood" by Taoists, the woman triggers the body's inner intelligence or instinct to redirect the blood to nourish and strengthen the sexual glands. Then the the entire body may be re-energized.

WARNING: When a woman's menstrual cycle does stop, pregnancy is not likely to occur during that time. Nevertheless, historical records show that whenever a woman discontinued the Deer Exercise, her menstrual cycle would resume, with the benefit of a prospect for a healthier pregnancy. For those women, stopping menstruation had no permanent effects. Women should not perform the Deer during pregnancy. The energy generated by the exercise combined with the accompanying increased stimulation of the sexual glands might induce premature labor.

INSTRUCTIONS FOR THE FEMALE DEER EXERCISE

As you do the two steps of this exercise, "feel" the fire or energy generate in your sexual glands and feel it rise upward along the spine into the breast and the head. (Never try to use visualization to help the energy rise. For reasons please refer to the section Instructions for the Male Deer Exercise.) Linking mind and body is a prerequisite for the harmonious and powerful functioning of vital energy. Bringing the energy to the pineal gland in the head is the Divine purpose.

Do this exercise in the morning upon rising and at night before retiring. If the appropriate time is not available, once a day will suffice.

First Stage:

1. Sit so that you can press the heal of one foot against the opening of your vagina. You will want a steady and fairly firm pressure against the clitoris. If it is not possible to place your foot in this position, then place a fairly hard, round object such as a baseball against the vaginal opening. (You may experience a pleasant sensation due to the stimulation of the genital area and the subsequent release of sexual energy.)

2. Rub your hands together vigorously. This will create heat in your hands by bringing the energy of your body into your palms and fingers.

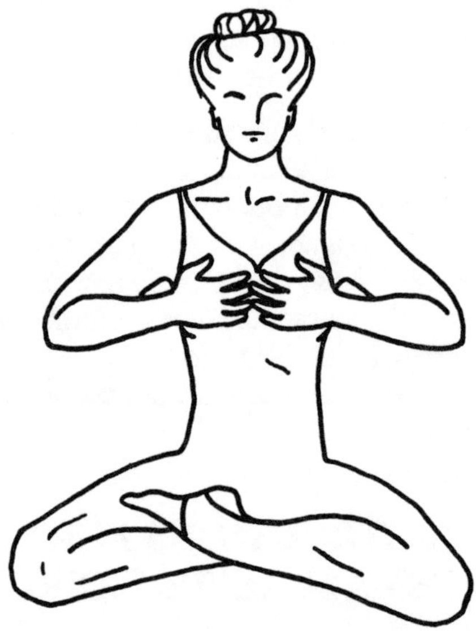

Figure 43. The Female Deer Exercise.

3. Place your hands on your breasts so that you feel the heat from your hands enter into the skin.

4. Rub your breasts slowly in outward, circular motions. Your right hand will turn counter-clockwise; your left, clockwise.

5. Rub in this circular manner for a minimum of thirty-six times or a maximum of 360 times *up* to two times a day. (Incidentally, it is not necessary to do 360 hand rotations once a woman has succeeded in stopping her period. Less than 100 rotations, up to twice a day, will suffice to maintain a suspension of menstruation once it has stopped. A woman is the best judge of when she should suspend or resume menstruation. Resumption occurs after cessation of the exercise.)

NOTE A: This outward circular rubbing motion of the hands is called *dispersion*, and helps to prevent or cure lumps and cancer of the breasts. One may reverse the motion of the hands to an inward rubbing motion. In this case the right hand circles in a clockwise fashion and the left hand circles counter-clockwise. This is called *stimulation* and its effect is to enlarge the breasts.

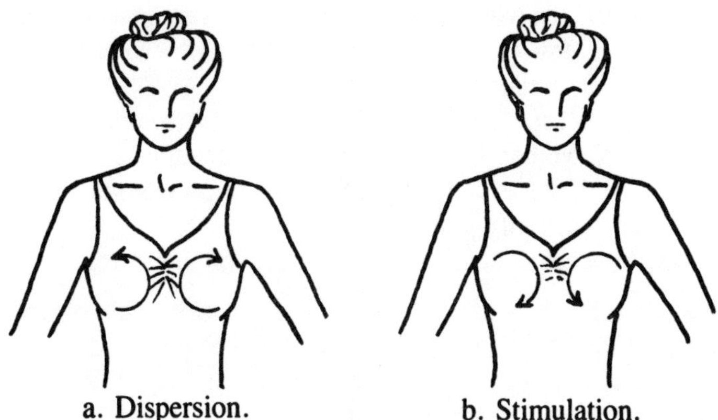

a. Dispersion. b. Stimulation.

Figures 44a and 44b. Dispersion and Stimulation.

Second Stage:

This exercise can be done sitting or lying down.

1. First tighten the muscles of your vagina and anus as if you were trying to close both openings, and then try to draw your rectum

upward inside the body, further contracting the anal muscles. When done properly this will feel as if air is being drawn up into your rectum and vagina. Hold these muscles tight for as long as you can comfortably.

2. Relax and repeat the anal and vaginal contractions. Do this as many times as you wish. The first few anal and vaginal contractions may be hard to do. Eventually, though, you will be able to increase the number of times you can do it as well as the length of time you are able to hold the contractions.

NOTE A: You may insert a finger into the vagina when you do the contractions, to determine the strength of your contractions.
NOTE B: The lips of the vagina are sensitive and must be massaged and stimulated during the Deer Exercise. Sitting on the heel of a foot or a ball serves this purpose. Finger pressure also serves this purpose.
NOTE C: If a woman finds it tiring to use both hands at once to do the breast rubbing, she can use one hand on the opposite breast while the other hand rests. Or, the free hand can be used to stimulate the vaginal opening in place of the heel. Another method is that the man rubs both breasts while the woman rubs or presses her vagina with her hand. As you can see, this is a very flexible exercise which can be adapted to individual preference.
NOTE D: When you practice the Deer, try to avoid touching the nipples. A woman's nipples are very sensitive and easily overstimulated. If the exercise is done correctly, a woman will notice an increased sensitivity in her nipples.
NOTE E: Always concentrate on what you are doing.

The same information in the previous section with regard to proper hygiene for men applies as well to women. The anus and genitals must be kept scrupulously clean and free from germs and feces. Please refer to the Sun Worship Exercise and other Internal Exercises which work to energize the anal and genital areas of the body.

When the exercise is done properly, a pleasant feeling will be felt to travel from the base of the anus through the spinal column to the top of the head. This is caused by the build-up of sexual energy and its movement up through the glandular system to the pineal gland and the top of the head. The feeling indicates that the exercise is working to rejuvenate the entire body, to preserve the body in perpetual youth.

It is crucial to learn control over the anal muscles if one is to master the later meditative and internal breathing exercises. These muscles may be described as a door or a lock. When shut in the female, as in the male, they close off the upper body and allow the energy to collect and build up in the abdominal channel. Without this build-up of energy, it is impossible to properly stimulate the sexual organs, and in turn, the other glands of the body. It is essential, then, to gain mastery over this lock if one is to strengthen one's system sufficiently to begin to energize the higher spiritual centers in the body.

PRONE POSITION FOR THE DEER EXERCISE

The prone position of the Deer may be used as an alternative when one is unable to practice the Deer in a sitting position.

1. Begin by lying on your left side. (Since the Deer is performed for only a short period of time, one may lie on either the right or left side without straining the heart.)

2. The left leg should be stretched straight out while the right leg, with the knee bent, lies on top. This position opens the pelvis so the anus and rectum may be contracted with ease.

3. The left arm lies on the floor with the hand down toward the left leg, and the right arm is placed, with the hand down, in front of the body. Support the head with a cushion so the neck does not become strained.

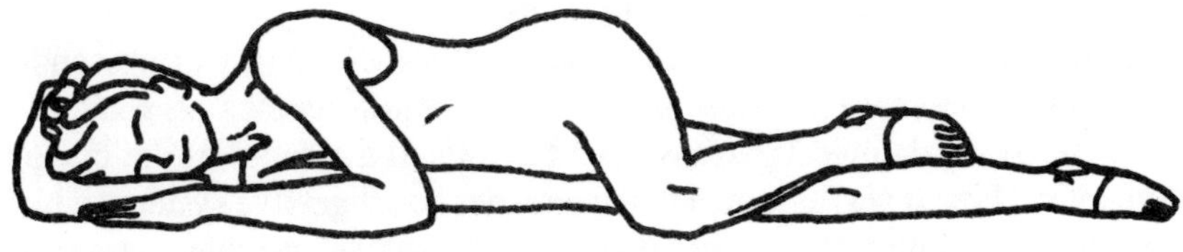

Figure 45. Prone Position for the Deer Exercise.

4. Perform the movements as outlined in the Deer Exercise. (One may forego the hand rubbing on the pubis if this is too uncomfortable. The main benefit of the Deer is gained from the tightening of the anal muscles.)

5. Combine the breathing as taught in the Crane Exercise to complete this pose. Repeat the breathing twelve times while simultaneously contracting the anal muscles.

NOTE: You may wish to practice this exercise while lying in the sunlight so that the sun bathes the anus and body in its health-enhancing and energy-producing light. Please refer ahead to the Sun Worship Exercise, which utilizes the energizing and germicidal qualities of the rays of the sun.

THE CRANE EXERCISE

A special species of crane can be found in China. These cranes—male and female—are distinguished by their poisonous red combs. The poisons which have been ingested throughout the crane's life are stored in its comb, causing the comb to be extremely poisonous. High-ranking soldiers of the early dynasties used this quality to demonstrate their loyalty to their princes. Those who were qualified to wear the combs around their necks or arms were so highly regarded that punishments for their wrongdoings were not meted out in the court of law; if these men did something wrong, they would commit suicide by licking the comb. The poisons stored in the comb were potent enough to kill a large man in minutes. Yet every bit of that poison passed through a crane's system without harming it. In fact, the red-combed crane was noted for its longevity.

In light of the crane's lethal diet—one composed mainly of poisonous amphibians and insects—the previous observation comes as a bit of a surprise. But past investigations have pinpointed the cause of the crane's longevity. First it was assumed that the cranes had digestive systems which were strong enough to take in lethal doses of toxins and then store them without harming the other organ systems. But it was found that their digestive systems did not differ markedly from those of other, poison-intolerant birds. So the ancient Taoists observing them determined there

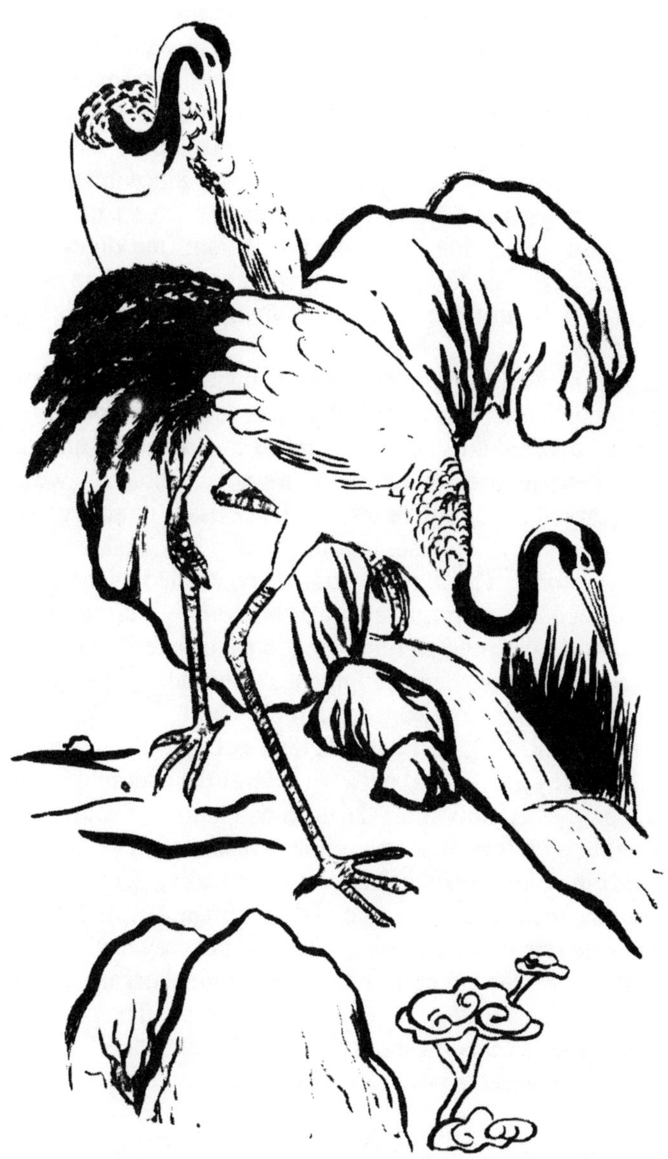

Illustration 4. The Crane.

was something else which gave them the ability to protect themselves from toxins. When those Taoists realized that the crane's unique pose—one leg folded into the belly and one leg holding the bird erect—gave the bird its unique characteristics, the Crane Exercise was developed.

As it stands, the crane will fold one leg into its belly and exert pressure on its abdominal muscles and internal organs, to stimulate and strengthen its digestive, respiratory and circulatory systems. This pose will not lose its efficaciousness when it is adapted for human use. Since human intestines are involuntary organs and are located in areas which are unreachable by external exercise, emulating the crane will benefit the digestive system greatly. Humans emulate the crane by practicing standing on one leg and then by learning to use the diaphragm to massage the digestive and intestinal organs.

Historically, as well as in modern times, man has suffered from many acute and chronic problems of the abdomen including constipation, diarrhea, ulcers, diverticulitis, and cancers of the stomach, intestines and colon. All of these diseases are caused by a similar problem—weakness in one or more parts of the digestive tract. When a tissue or an organ is weak, it is more susceptible to disease, and the greater the weakness, the more intense the symptoms. The digestive tract is controlled by the involuntary muscles. We need, then, to find a way to bring these muscles and organs under our control. We need to force the stomach, intestines and colon to move, to work so they may be strengthened. Normally, when we breathe, the lungs tend to expand outward toward the chest. The Crane Exercise, however, forces the lungs downward, and because the intestines have nowhere to go, they are pressed outward against the abdominal muscles to form a little ball. This motion breaks up constipation, encourages absorption of nutrients, and strengthens the entire digestive tract while stimulating the lungs and circulatory system. In this way, invading germs do not have a good environment in which to settle and germinate because one's bowel movements are so strong and regular. Then it is not easy to get diseases.The Crane also increases the circulation to the abdominal organs and muscles. Thus, it can reduce cholesterol and fat accumulation. The pose also helps asthma through its effects on the lungs, and because the lungs and skin work together as a unit, the pose can help skin disorders such as rashes and sores.

Poor breathing habits are a major cause of weakness and disease in the body. One tends to breathe using only the upper half of the lungs and only rarely does one utilize the lower portion of the lungs. (Autopsies have sometimes shown that the middle and lower lobes of the lungs have never even been used. They are either like new or atrophied.) The stale air that remains in the lower areas of the lungs and the warm moisture which accompanies the stale air provide the conditions necessary for germs to flourish. Also, the air we breathe contains Chi, or energy, in addition to oxygen, nitrogen, carbon, etc. We depend on the air we breathe not only to give us oxygen, which is necessary for our metabolism, but also to provide us with energy, the electrical charge without which we will quickly weaken and die. Poor breathing habits also encompass fast breathing. Such breathing is violent, and it damages the delicate membranes and increases the rate of the heart beat. It also prevents us from getting the necessary nourishment for the air we inhale. Any number of problems, such as disease, headache, indigestion, dizziness, poor blood circulation, and aging can arise. (The aging process is hastened when the heart rate increases. The rate goes up as stress and tension mount. Later, signs of age show up on the face as stress and tension effectively choke cell nourishment.)

We want, therefore, to correct poor breathing habits. Slow diaphragmatic breathing, as taught in the Crane, allows for full expansion of the lungs and full absorption of energy from the air intake, all the while exercising the lungs and gently massaging the internal organs. The Crane also encourages us to improve our circulation and lower the heart rate at the same time. (The ideal rate is 45 beats/minute, the rate the heart sinks down to during sleep.)

In sum, the Crane Exercise is designed to strengthen the organs within the trunk of the body. Even though these organs are controlled by the autonomic, or involuntary, nervous system, the Crane enables us to balance the energy and thereby promote a smoother functioning of these organs.

INSTRUCTIONS FOR THE CRANE EXERCISE

This pose may be practiced while standing, sitting, or while lying down on your back.

1. Begin by rubbing the palms of your hands together vigorously. This creates heat in your hands and brings the energy of your body into your palms and fingers.

2. Place your hands, palms down, on your lower abdomen so that they lie on either side of your navel.

3. Keeping your mouth closed, inhale through your nostrils.

4. Begin to exhale slowly, while pressing your hands down lightly so that the abdomen forms a hollow cavity. This motion gently forces the air out of the lower lungs. (In this instance, the hands are like the leg of the crane.) As you do part four of the exercise, imagine that every drop of air is leaving the lungs and that as it leaves the microorganisms are carried out also.

5. After you have exhaled completely, slowly inhale again. As you inhale, extend your abdomen outward so that it becomes like a balloon. Try not to allow the chest to expand—use only the muscles in your lower abdomen.

6. One complete exhalation, followed by an inhalation, constitutes one round of breathing. At first you will probably only be able to do two or three rounds of breathing at one sitting. Gradually you will be able to increase the number until you have reached 12 rounds.

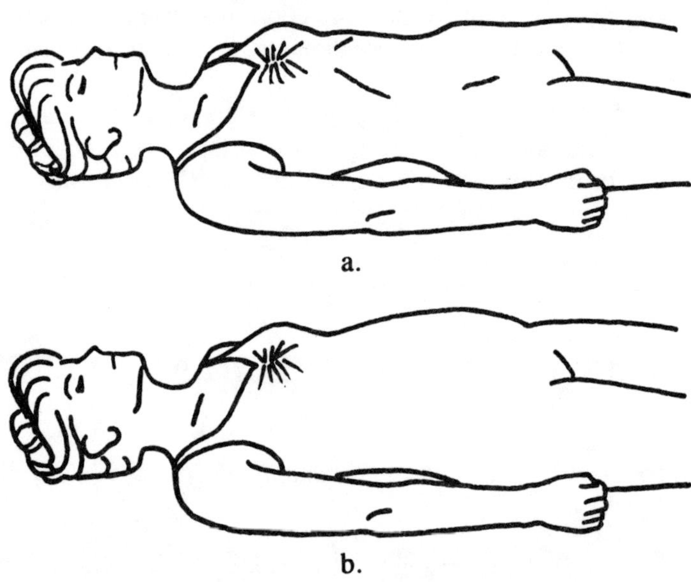

Figures 46a and 46b. The Crane Exercise.

NOTE A: It is not necessary to force either the inhalation or the exhalation. With continued practice you will be able to extend and contract your abdomen quite easily while breathing very slowly. In the beginning your hands act as guides to help you learn the exercise. Once you have learned the breathing, it is not necessary to continue using your hands. Breathing must be very slow. So slow, in fact, that a hair in front of the nose will not move either during inhalation or exhalation.

NOTE B: Once you have mastered the Crane Exercise, you may combine the anal lock as described in the Deer Exercise with the Crane breathing. This will increase the strength of the exercise.

NOTE C: Always concentrate on what you are doing.

NOTE D: Women should not perform the Crane Exercise during pregnancy as the in and out motions of the abdomen may create unpleasant feelings within the abdomen.

The best time to do the Crane Exercise is in the morning, while facing the sun, if possible. As you inhale, feel the energy of the sun come into your body, and feel as you exhale the toxins and wastes leave your body.

When done before retiring at night, the Crane Exercise gives a gentle massage to the inner organs which helps calm the body, relaxing it for proper and restful sleep.

One organ which benefits greatly from the Crane is the lung. As it is one of the three filter systems of the body—it filters out gaseous wastes and carbon dioxide—it must function perfectly for good health. The simplest way to good respiratory and circulatory health is through nourishing, relaxing, and comforting breathing. The Crane will help us re-learn this kind of breathing, as it was once used naturally when we were babies. Except for singers, most of us lose this knowledge as we grow older.

Eventually you will want to learn to do the Crane breathing so slowly that one breath will take you 10 minutes to complete. Many people have more trouble taking long inhalations than long exhalations, but with training both can be done. In accomplishing this, we learn to control every cell in our bodies, to help it follow the mind. Achieving this first stage will facilitate the our progress to next stage, wherein every mental movement follows the way of God.

Like the Deer Exercise, the Crane must be mastered as it is also the basis for future meditative and advanced breathing techniques.

THE STANDING CRANE

This exercise is similar to the sitting Crane Exercise, only it is performed while standing. It helps develop balance, stimulates the nervous system, strengthens the inner organs, and increases the flexibility of the knee, ankle, and hip joints. It also increases the circulation in the legs and feet and reverses tendencies toward cramps in the legs and feet, varicose veins, and cold feet.

1. Stand with your feet together, toes and heels touching.
2. Pick up one foot and rub the sole of that foot on the opposite calf.

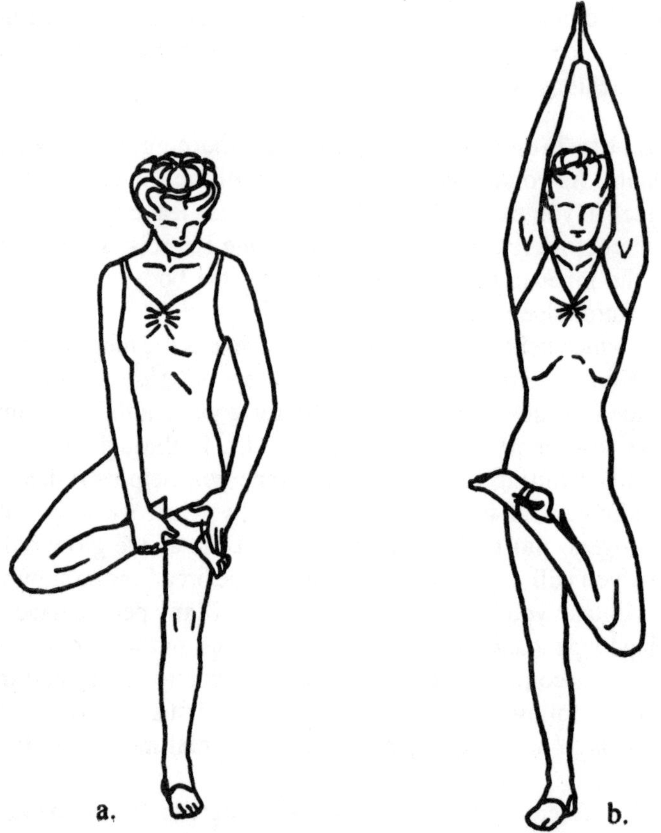

Figure 47a and 47b. The Standing Crane.

3. Gradually work your foot up the leg, stopping every few inches or so to continue the rubbing motion, until your foot rests on the outside thigh of your opposite leg. The heel will be in toward the pelvis, and the toes will extend past the thigh near the hip joint.

4. Now massage the sole of your foot with your hands and manipulate the toes to stimulate the nerves and circulation in your foot.

5. Then slowly raise your arms over your head sideways as you inhale, and bring your palms as close together as possible.

6. Breathing normally, balance in this position for as long as you feel comfortable.

7. Exhaling, lower your arms and foot and repeat the exercise with your other foot.

8. Do this exercise once with each foot.

It may not be possible to balance in the full position at first, but with continued practice the pose will open up, and you will find yourself performing it with ease. The increased ability to balance will have enormous beneficial effects on your everyday life.

SOLAR PLEXUS EXERCISE

The ancient Taoists believed that the human body was controlled and operated by two brains instead of one. Besides the familiar brain in the head, there is also a "brain" in the abdomen. We know that the entire body is operated by nerves. But whenever the subject of nerves is brought up, we invariably link in the cerebral brain while never venturing further beyond that point. The ancient Taoists went one step further by linking the nervous system to another "brain" and maintaining that that nervous center existed in the abdomen and was at least equal in importance to the cerebral brain.

The modern anatomical term for this abdominal nervous center is "solar plexus". A mass of nerve cells, the solar plexus is found in the center of the torso, beneath the heart and behind the stomach. Being in closer proximity to the abdominal organs than the cerebral brain, the solar plexus has nerves radiating out directly to the organs. One can say that the relationship of the solar plexus to the abdominal organs is even more direct and intimate than that of the cerebral brain. That is why Taoists call the solar plexus the "abdominal brain".

Responsibility for maintaining and balancing internal organ functions lies in the abdominal brain. Its presence can be clearly felt when a person in daily life feels anger, happiness, distress, sorrow, love, hate, and other emotions, all arising from within the internal organs. Feelings arise when an organ is disturbed or dysfunctioning, but they are felt at the solar plexus and later surface as physiological reactions. When a feeling is generated, the solar plexus must reestablish balance among the organs and correct organ dysfunctions—a struggle that can be painfully felt at the solar plexus.

In the minds of Taoists, the generation and sensation of feelings are functions of the abdominal area, not the cerebral brain. The cerebral brain is like a library where all data (life experience, education, knowledge, etc.) is stored. In modern terms, it functions exactly like a computer center.

The function of the solar plexus actually involves every organ in the abdomen. To the Taoist, excitement is related to the heart; anger, liver; worry, spleen-pancreas; sorrow, lungs; and fear, kidney. According to the Five Element Theory, excessive excitement hurts the small intestines, sexual organs, heart and blood vessels; excessive anger, the nervous system, liver and gallbladder; excessive worry or consideration, muscle tone, stomach and spleen-pancreas; excessive sorrow or sadness, the lungs, large intestines, skin and hair; excessive fear, the bones, kidneys and bladder. This is not to say that feelings are bad for the organs. They are God-given antagonists that temper the solar plexus. And when the solar plexus benefits, everything else along the cyclical chain of influence, including the organs, benefits. Therefore, if the internal organs are healthy and balanced, the feelings will naturally be balanced and peaceful. Peaceful feelings cannot be forced by thoughts or reasoning from the cerebral brain. Peaceful attitudes come from internal peace, not thoughts.

When the solar plexus is healthy, organs can immediately recover from stress and tension and resume proper functioning. It is when its balance is lost that the following problems arise: insomnia, hypertension, cardiovascular diseases, heart weakness, heart attack, stroke, chronic bronchitis, duodenal infection, ulcer, gastroenteritis, gastritis, constipation, diarrhea, lack of absorption (small intestine), menstruational cramps and related problems, impotence, etc.

How can the balance of the solar plexus be lost? According to the

Two-Brain Theory of Taoism, normal newborn babies have more abdominal brain functions than cerebral brain functions. Their cerebral brains are blank, without information that adults deem critical for survival, yet they hardly ever suffer from the health problems that plague or kill adults. With gradual absorption of living experience and artificial education, their cerebral brains gradually develop. Because some cultures value huge memory stores of facts and subsequently stress continuous cerebral (rational) development over inner development (true feeling), the abdominal brain functions are gradually forgotten or surpressed. Then the results of this direction of emphasis are a great library of recorded information (the cerebral brain gets bigger and bigger) and a great succession of physical and mental problems, the so called modern diseases listed above. In other words, human beings, in denying their true feelings, are misguidedly cutting off the functions of their solar plexus, causing their organs to become inoperative, and shortening their lives. The basic outward sign of an atrophied solar plexus and its associated ailments is a distended belly. The accumulation of dead cells, waste, and fatty tissues indicates that the solar plexus is in one of the various stages of atrophy. The distended belly and its hidden ailments are never seen in lively young children.

True feelings are centered at the solar plexus, not the brain. The brain records only the memory of a feeling. Misguidedly, we are taught to use our powers of reason—that is, cerebral rationality—to suppress our feelings. In suppressing our feelings, we suppress the solar plexus from functioning. According to a law of physics, where there is greatest pressure, there is greatest likelihood of explosion. If we keep suppressing, the physical and psychological time bombs we have set will explode, and all that we have been striving for (a cold rational head and its supposedly attendant successes) will be lost. When the organs that give the body life become inoperative, the facts that have been stored in the brain get jumbled and confused, burying true wisdom and intelligence. Looking at today's society we know that using rational to suppress feeling is useless. In truth it has created more physically and psychologically unhealthy individuals than ever before.

According to Taoism, using rational to suppress true feeling is not the solution. In the *Tao Te Ching*, chapter 55, Lao-Tse said that "in order to attain health and longevity, man must learn to return to his infancy". The salient point is that the abdominal brain must be developed in order to recapture or maintain youth. At least both brains must be developed in balance. This is achieved through the following steps: 1. Balancing the organs according to the Five Element Theory, and 2. Strengthening the abdominal brain so that it could handle more emotional pressure. This is most different from most educational and religious teachings, but this is one of the greatest secrets of Taoism.

Most religions and regular educational institutions teach people to suppress feeling with reasoning, logic, and rationality. Artificial reasoning appears to be logical, reasonable, and objective at first glance, and it is easily programmed into the cerebral brain. But when a complicated and complex case occurs, it may not be truly appropriate in subjective situations. So proper guidance cannot be found. Instead, one finds only confusion and frustration. That is why one often hears people speak of the conflict between their hearts and minds. One can only find proper guidance if one looks into one's own deep and true feelings.

According to Taoism, correct feelings—that is, peaceful feelings—always come with healthy and balanced internal organ functions. If one organ is over-active, it can be difficult to reach peace or proper guidance.

In this book, many exercises are provided that provide techniques to develop and balance the internal organs and subsequently the two brains, but the Crane Exercise and its many variations are the most direct in serving this purpose.

Some meditators teach people to slow down the cerebral brain to reduce stress and tension. Meditation has the effect of temporarily stopping cerebral reasoning. Recently, many organizations recognized stress and tension as the great enemy of its members, and recommended meditation programs for saving their health. But there are those who are so overwhelmed by too many attachments and desires—their brains have been programmed to race for too long—that they are unable to slow their brains down. If these people were placed in a meditation program and forced to slow down their brains, the results would be disastrous. Forcing a different direction upon the brain creates more confusion and causes illusions and frustration, finally resulting in worsening conditions of stress and tension. At worst, this can lead to a case of schizophrenia.

Even if meditation were done properly to reduce stress and tension, it would not naturally strengthen the solar plexus, and a two-brain balance can never be reached.

If a side-effect free method for strengthening the solar plexus exists that naturally reduces stress and tension (not by slowing down the cerebral brain) and balances both brains at the same time, then the Solar Plexus Exercise would be the only and perfect answer. The original Taoist term for the Solar Plexus Exercise translates into English as, "The Fire Burns the Wheel". The "Fire" means feeling, and the "Wheel" means solar plexus. According to the ancients, this exercise strengthens the true feelings in the abdominal cavity. Building up this "fire" will help "burn out" every disease associated with this area of the body, including diarrhea, constipation, flatulence, diverticulitis, cancer, and other disorders.

To avoid overloading your cerebral brain, it is best to recognize these few early warning signs: headache, stiff neck, stiff shoulder, confusion, illusions, forgetfullness, or spaciness. Headaches indicate mental overload, which in turn indicates that the cerebral brain is out of balance with respect to the abdominal brain. Neck/shoulder stiffness indicates that the nerves closest to the cerebral brain are unable to handle the overload from it. Whenever the above symptoms arise, do the following exercise. It will help temporary as well as long term problems resulting from cerebral-abdominal imbalance.

This exercise can be done anywhere, anytime.

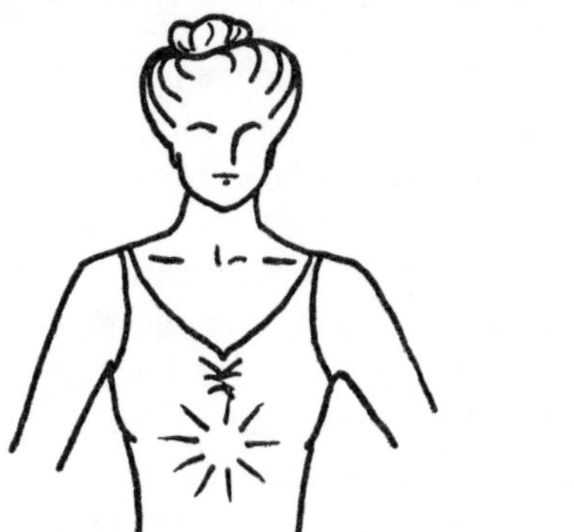

Figure 48. The Solar Plexus.

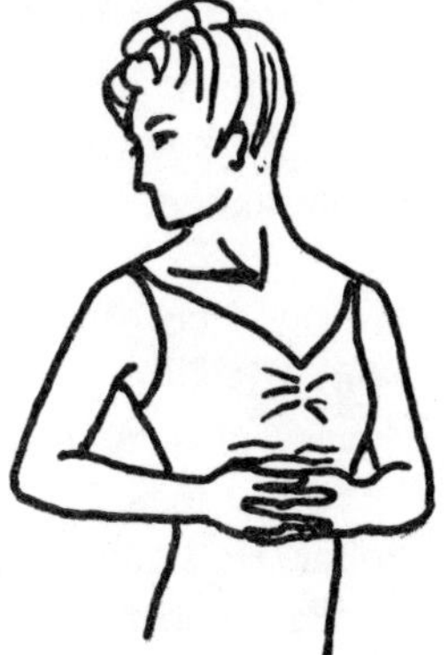

Figure 49. The Solar Plexus Exercise.

1. While sitting or standing, place both hands on your stomach. Face front and inhale and feel the air expand your stomach.

2. Then exhale. As you exhale, use your hands to push in and up your stomach. As you execute these motions, turn your upper torso and head slowly toward your left side as far as possible and look to your left. Meanwhile twist your pelvis to the right.

3. Inhale and bring your entire body back into alignment, facing front. As you do this, let your hands release your stomach slowly until

they are resting gently on the skin surface.

4. Exhale again. But as you exhale, turn your upper torso and head slowly to the right side. Look to your right. Meanwhile push your stomach in and up again as you twist your pelvis to the left.

5. While inhaling, bring your body back into alignment, facing front. Repeat this exercise 4 to 36 times.

NOTE A: How many times you are able to do the exercise depends on the condition of your neck and shoulders. If you experience stiffness and pain at the neck and shoulders, do small repetitions until the condition clears. Then you may increase the repetitions in increments.

NOTE B: When you do the exercise, concentrate on the solar plexus area, which is located under the heart and behind the stomach. The more you concentrate, the more benefits you gain from the exercise.

The placing of the hands on the abdomen helps concentration, and the turning of the neck relaxes the nerves in the neck, shoulder, and cerebral brain. As you can see, the exercise is designed to balance both brains in one movement.

One day the vice president of a famous university came in seeking consultation. His situation correlated exactly with that caused by brain overuse; every ailment listed earlier afflicted him. He had undergone surgery several times for abdominal problems. Half of his liver was nonfunctional. He lived on tranquilizers. And because of the blood pressure pills, pills for heart disease, pills for insomnia, and so on, he became a pill bottle. He was, by his own admission, like a zombie, half dead physically and mentally. I recommended the Solar Plexus Exercise for his afflictions. About a week later he came back. He said he did not trust the simplicity of the exercise at first, because his condition had lasted for many, many years and was lately worsening week by week, but he faithfully practiced it nevertheless for one week. When 50% of his symptoms disappeared, he became a believer, although his doctor could not believe what happened. A few days later, his doctor called me to ask what method, shots or pills I used on his patient to get such results. When I told him what his patient used, the doctor said, "Excuse me . . . I would never believe it." Two months later, I learned that the executive had become like a college student; he had played ball with a few students. To celebrate his new life, he held a party. There he introduced me and held up my hand and said, "This is my saviour!" He was still very healthy seven years later, though he "never touched another pill".

THE TURTLE

Ancient Taoist texts tell the story of a family which escaped to the hills during a time of war. They took up residence in a cave deep within the mountains. One day, a part of the mountain crashed down, sealing the family within the cave. No amount of digging from inside could free them, so they sat to await the chance that someone would discover their plight. Months passed, as the family anxiously awaited their death due to their dwindling supply of food. One day, they discovered a turtle which had been in the cave with them from the beginning. The turtle had been so still that they had earlier mistaken it for a rock. Now they studied it with the utmost fascination, wondering how it had been able to survive until now. As they observed it over the following days, they found the only movements it made were to extend and shrink its head in and out of its shell. Occasionally, it would stop to catch on its tongue a drop of water which had fallen from the ceiling. It had no other sustenance. Soon the family was out of food. Facing starvation, with nothing else to guide them, they began to imitate the movements of the turtle in hopes the simple exercise would somehow keep them alive. Many years passed before others discovered the family and removed the boulders which had blocked their escape. When the records were checked, it was found that 800 years had passed since the time the family had first been locked in the cave! News of their survival soon spread and their fellow countrymen were astonished on learning that only a few drops of water and a simple exercise imitating the movements of a tortoise had sustained them through the centuries.

You may not believe this story, and it is recited only to encourage people to follow the Turtle Exercise, but the Turtle pose is one which stimulates the nerves. It stretches, stimulates, and energizes all the nerves of the neck which lead to the brain and to the lower extremities of the body. The neck forms the central pathway for all the nerves leading to and from the brain through the central nervous system. If we are able to gain control over this complex of nerves, we will control the entire functioning of the body. We can cut off an arm and remain alive, but we cannot cut off our heads and still expect to live; therefore, we must recognize the importance of exercising the area of the neck, as it increases the circulation and carries away deposits which would otherwise impair the proper functioning of the nerves, tissues, arteries and veins of the neck.

The Turtle stretches the entire spine, energizes the neck, strengthens the shoulder muscles, and removes tiredness, stiffness and soreness from the neck and shoulder muscles. In addition, the thyroid and parathyroid glands are stimulated and strengthened, improving the body's metabolism. If one performs the Turtle on a daily basis, one will feel younger and radiate an inner beauty which comes only through the proper functioning of one's inner energy systems.

INSTRUCTIONS FOR THE TURTLE EXERCISE

This exercise may be done standing or sitting. The best time to perform the exercise is in the early morning upon rising, and just before retiring at night. It may also be practiced any time you feel tension or tightness in the neck or upper back and shoulders.

1. Bring your chin down onto your chest. At the same time stretch the

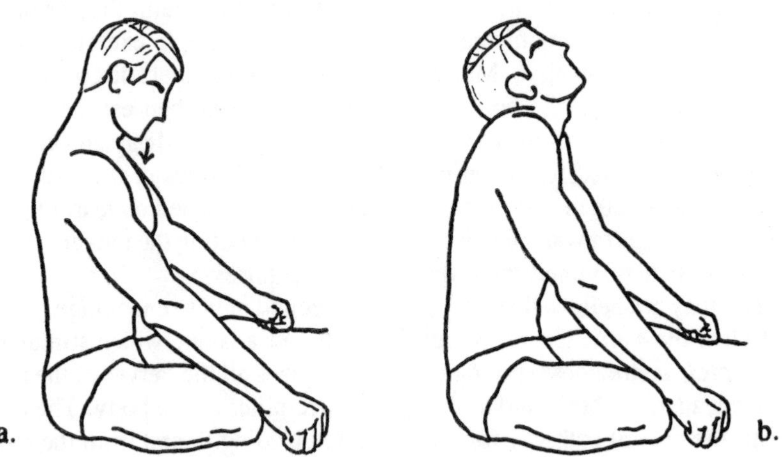

Figures 50a and 50b. The Turtle Exercise.

top of your head upward. Slowly inhale as you do this. The back of your neck will feel an upward pull and your shoulders will relax downward.

2. Slowly bring the back of your skull down, as if to touch it on the back of your neck. Slowly exhale as you do this movement. Your chin will be pulled upward, and your throat will be slightly stretched. Also, your shoulders will be pulled upward on either side of your head, as if you were trying to touch them to your ears.

3. Repeat this cycle for a total of 12 times, taking care not to force the movements.

NOTE A: You may find it helpful to synchronize the movements of the Turtle with the breathing techniques of the Crane. In this case, as you stretch the head upward, inhale; as you bring the head down and lift the chin up, exhale. In any case, please proceed slowly.

NOTE B: While doing the Turtle Exercise, look straight ahead at a soft or muted light, or keep the eyes gently closed. You want to hold the rest of the body relaxed and keep the fingers clasped around the thumbs as you make a fist. This hand lock prevents energy from spilling out through the fingers.

NOTE C: Always remember to concentrate on what you are doing. If the mind wanders, bring it gently back.

Patience in practicing this exercise will lead you to a treasure of healthful, emotional, and spiritual benefits. Upon performing the pose correctly, you may immediately feel a diminishing of any tension or tiredness in the neck or upper back.

COMBINING THE DEER, CRANE, AND TURTLE EXERCISES

Once one is able to comfortably practice the three foundation exercises on an individual basis, then the Deer, Crane, and Turtle may be put together and performed as one basic exercise. This is accomplished by combining the component parts of each exercise into one single exercise. Basically, one will synchronize the neck stretching as learned in the Turtle with the breathing as taught in the Crane, together with the anal lock and hand rubbing as taught in the Deer (eventually the hand rubbing may be discontinued and only the anal lock used). This may seem a bit confusing when first practiced, but if one has become proficient in the individual exercises before putting them together, it should not take long to master this combination technique.

Each of the three exercises, as well as the combination technique when mastered, should be practiced daily, preferably once in the morning and again at night for optimum benefits. If one were only to practice these three basic exercises, one's health would expand a great deal. The Crane will strengthen and stimulate the circulatory and digestive systems. If these two complexes are strong, then it will not be easy to accumulate weakness and disease. The Deer stimulates the physical as well as the spiritual being of the practitioner. It improves one's sexual energy and ensures a balanced glandular and hormonal system. It is said that if one has strong sexual glands, one may never grow old. The Turtle energizes the nerves and strengthens the brain, spinal column, and neck region. Possessing a strong central nervous system helps balance one's mental energy and eventually helps to bring peace of mind.

Every human being is a meld of three bodies: a physical body, a mental body, and a spiritual body. The physical body houses the basic needs for sex, violence, food, and entertainment. The mental body houses the emotions, thoughts, and will. The spiritual body houses intuition, conscience, and illumination—or communication with God.

The proper sequence of influence between these three forces should be thus: the physical body functions only to bring into fruition the plans formulated in the mental body, and the mental body formulates plans only in accordance to spiritual laws. A society functioning under such an order of influence would be free of all evils and ills.

However, this is often not so. Since Adam ate of the forbidden fruit in the Garden of Eden, the order of influence has been turned upside down. The body's needs overpower the guidance of the spirit, and the mind becomes the body's agent. The result was chaos.

We need, then, to bring the mind back, to return to the natural order. The Deer, Crane, and Turtle Exercises help us do so gently and pleasantly, by freeing us from the body's needs.

Taoist teachings are very practical. They teach that we are each responsible for our own state of being—physical, mental and emotional, as well as spiritual. It is for the purpose of realizing these truths that the Internal

Exercises were developed.

THE SITTING POSITION

Taoist teachings offer correct methods for sitting, standing, walking, and lying down. People tend to sacrifice much of their everyday energy in supporting unhealthy forms of posture. The following suggestions provide simple ways of arranging our bodies so that we enhance rather than retard the natural flow of energy as we go about our daily lives.

Sitting correctly increases one's energy and improves the health of the body even as one sits. It is best for everyone to sit with the heel of one foot pressed tightly against the perineum. For the male, the heel will press against the prostate; for the female, the heel will press against the clitoris. The other leg may be kept extended or brought upon the opposite leg to form the half-lotus position. If neither of these positions is comfortable, you may use an object such as a hard ball to create the pressure. Remember always to keep your spine as straight as possible. You may also practice locking your sphincter muscles around the anus while in this position, but understand that keeping the anus locked all the time will result in too much tension in the body, causing a negative reaction. You need to observe

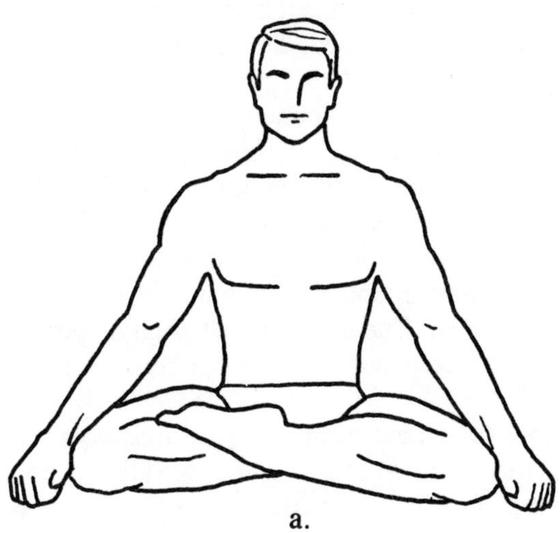

a.

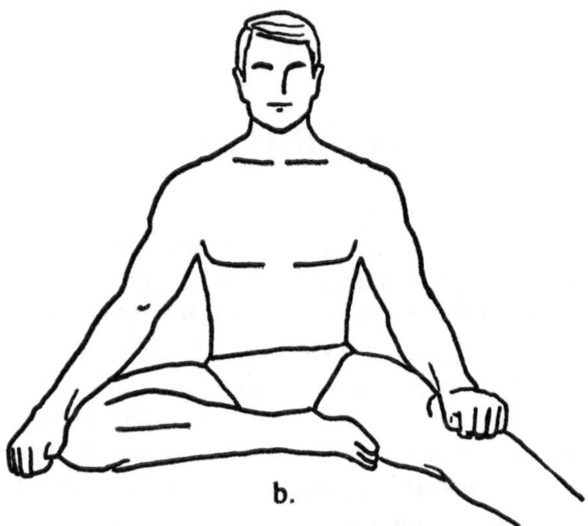

Figures 51a and 51b. Sitting Positions.

moderation in all these exercises. There need never be strain or overexertion to obtain maximum benefits from the Internal Exercises.

This sitting position opens the pelvis so that the heel may be pressed comfortably into the perineum. Through overuse of the sexual organs, we lose a great deal of energy. Even through inactivity the sexual organs may grow weak. Since the sexual organs are the basic glands in the body, they need to be protected and energized. This sitting position protects against the loss of energy through the "energy gate" (prostate or clitoris) and enables you to build up additional energy in your sexual glands.

When sitting on a chair or couch, keep your thighs parallel to the floor with your spine erect. This is the healthiest position for regular sitting. You do not want a chair to be so high that your feet have difficulty touching the ground, nor so low that your knees are above your thighs. Sitting back in a plush sofa may seem comfortable at first, but it promotes poor posture and is not a healthy way to sit. The bones do not align properly, the vertebrae become crooked, and your energy does not flow correctly through the spinal column.

The two methods for correct sitting are to be used whenever you practice the Internal Exercises—including the breathing and meditation techniques—as well as when you work at a desk, converse with someone, or read a book. Sitting properly promotes a healthy flow of energy in your body and keeps your mind in an alert and responsive state.

THE STANDING POSITION

When standing, keep your feet shoulder-width apart and parallel to each other. Your weight should be evenly distributed along your feet. Too much weight on the heels will throw your spine off center, make your abdomen sag, stimulate too many nerves in your heels, and make your brain lazy. This position keeps your mind alert and will give you a feeling of lightness in your body.

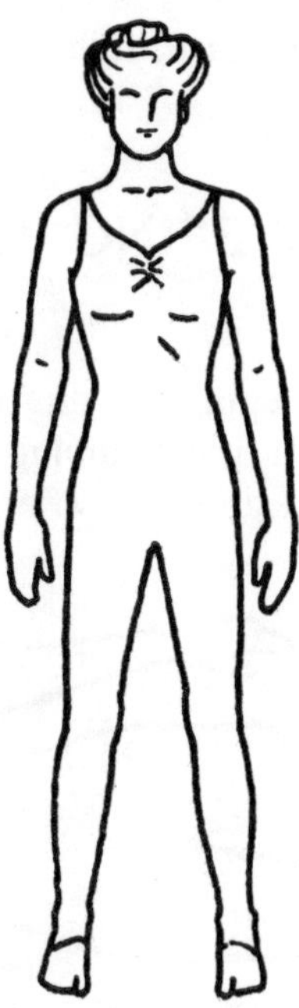

Figure 52. Standing Position.

WALKING

When walking, never hurry, lest you build up an excessive amount of tension and make the heart beat too rapidly. It is better not to run unless necessary. Leave early for your destination to avoid needless stress and tension; stress is perhaps the biggest enemy of the body. When you are rushed in your activities, there is a build-up of unnecessary tension. Over a period of time, this may lead to weakness and to diseases such as cancers and ulcers.

While walking, your steps should be even, and only the legs should be used so that your mind remains alert and peaceful. Always walk with complete attention to, and awareness of, what you are doing. Walk at a constant speed, not too fast or too slow, but at just an easy gait. The feet should be parallel to each other, with the heels and toes pointing straight ahead. When you walk correctly, you will feel like you are walking on a cloud: your steps will be balanced, light, and airy.

THE SLEEPING POSITION

The best position for sleeping is lying on your back. Many people experience nightmares when first assuming this sleeping position. However, the nightmares should disappear after a little while. The next best

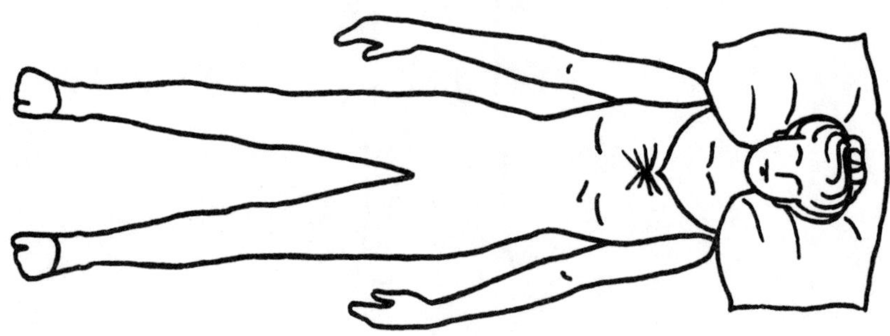

Figure 53. Sleeping Position.

position is to lie on your right side. If you lie on your left side, the lungs, stomach, and liver will press into your heart. This additional weight strains the heart and may be a factor in causing heart disease. Also avoid sleeping on your stomach. This puts an excessive amount of pressure on the lungs, heart, and internal organs; produces shallow breathing habits; and often results in severe neck strain and pain due to the head and neck being twisted.

Try to sleep in a well-ventilated room, preferably with your head to the north and your feet to the south so you are in line with the natural flow of energy on the planet. Avoid oversleeping as this makes the body sluggish and promotes weakness. Too little sleep causes this also. Between seven and eight hours of sleep is sufficient for the average person. If you need more than that, it may be that your system has been weakened by improper exercise, diet, or living habits.

HEAD RUBBING EXERCISE

This is an excellent exercise for stimulating the circulation in the scalp and preventing the hair from falling out, because the hair follicles become nourished with the added circulation.

1. Press your hands on the points of the head indicated in figure 54a. Do not scratch these points, simply rub the skin back and forth without moving your hands from your head.

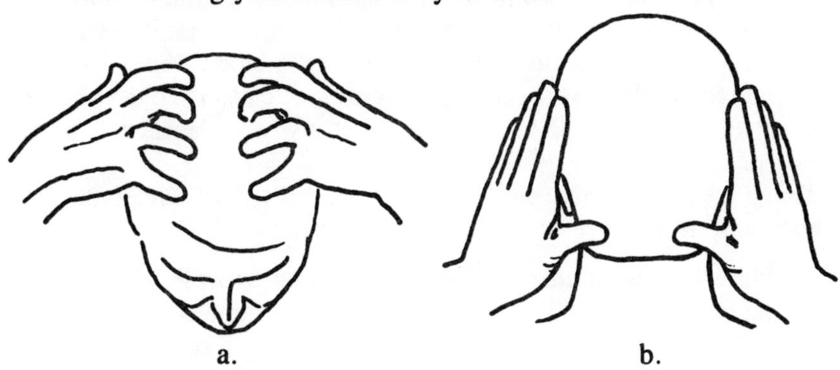

Figures 54a and 54b. Head Rubbing.

2. Press your fingers into the points on the back of your neck as indicated in figure 54b. Press in and rub at the same time. This exercise removes tension and fatigue from the upper back and neck and removes or prevents tension headaches.

THE EYE EXERCISES

The eyes are the openings to the liver. People who suffer from eye problems usually suffer from liver disorders and vice-versa. As anger is a symptom of liver dysfunction in Taoist theory, people who use their eyes too much may become angry. The Internal Exercises for the eyes will strengthen both the eyes and the liver and help such serious disorders as cataracts, astigmatism, nearsightedness, glaucoma, and liver problems.

The eyes, specifically their movements, are indicative of an individual's intelligence. People who are clever have large eye movements and are always exploring their environment. Slow eye movement or a lack of eye movement indicates a repressed level of intelligence, which may also be helped through stimulation of the eyes.

Poor blood circulation, indicated by dark circles under the eyes, can also be helped by doing the Eye Exercises. Poor blood circulation results from long periods of inactivity, such as those spent in front of a television set. Often the first signs of sluggish circulation are chilly sensations, which result when the body temperature rises above room temperature, causing the surroundings to be cooler than the body. Like car engines, our bodies need cool liquids to circulate through them and remove heat. If circulation is sluggish, body temperature goes up. Then the blood "boils", forms skins, and forms clots. So in order to prevent blood clots, the Eye and other Internal Exercises should be done, especially when television is being watched.

Doing the Eye Exercise can also help bags or puffiness under the eyes which indicate water retention or bad metabolism.

1. Place thumbs on rim of the eye sockets at the upper inside corner of the eyes. There is a slight depression in the bone at the correct point. Those points are designated by the letter A in figure 55a. Press in deeply. Any pain indicates some blockage. Then massage the points for a count of 10. Release. Repeat for a total of 3 times.

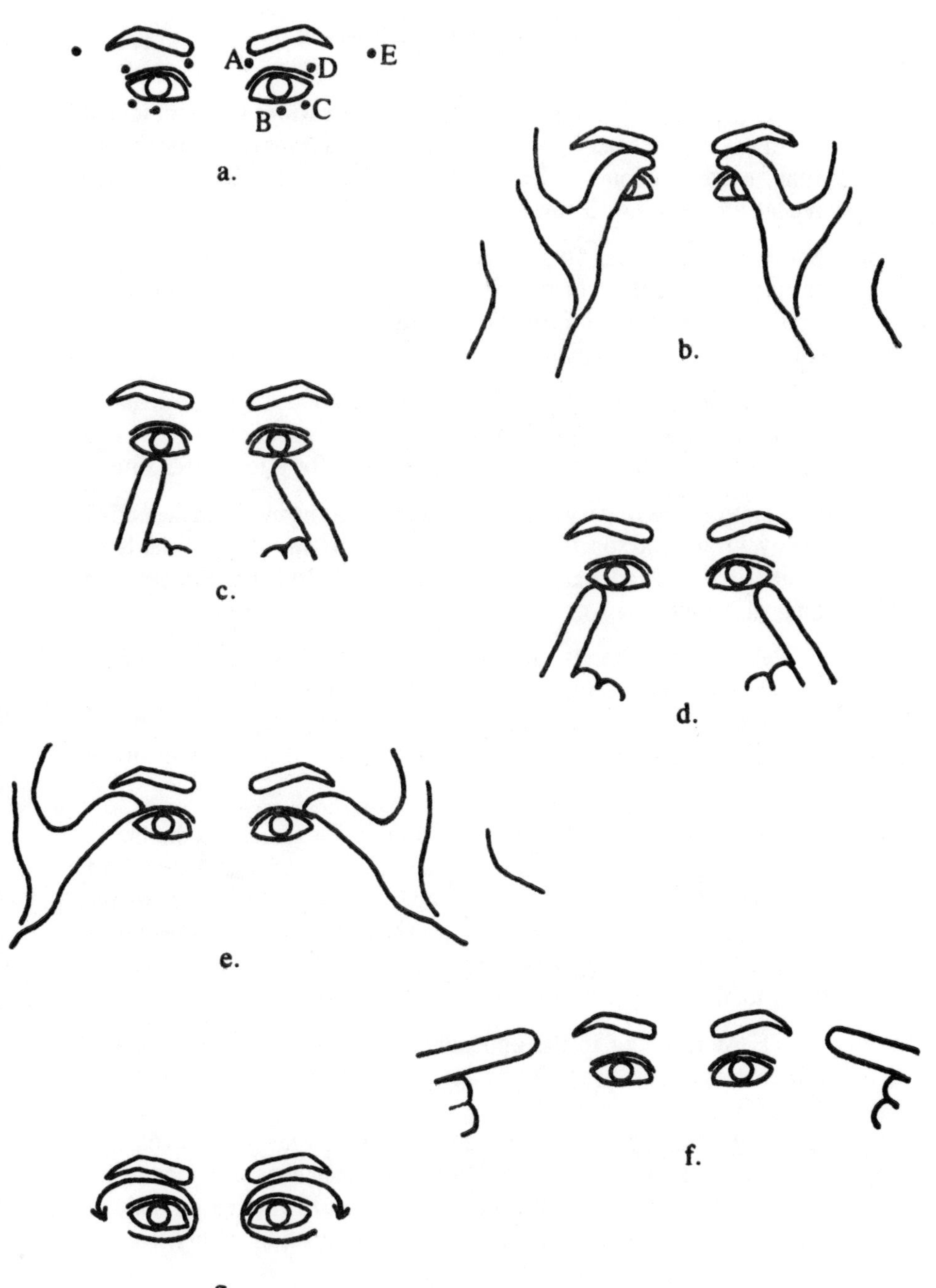

Figures 55a — 55g. Eye Exercises.

2. Next, place index fingers in the small depressions at the middle of the lower eye sockets—points designated by B. Press in deeply on the rims, not cheekbones. Massage for a count of 10. Release. Then repeat for a total of 3 times.

3. Then, place index fingers on lower eye socket 1/4 of the distance from outside corners of the eyes. (Look for letter C in figure 55d.) Press and massage for a count of 10. Release. Repeat for a total of 3 times.

4. Place middle fingers on top of eye sockets about 1/3 of the distance from the outside corners of the eyes. (Look for letter D.) Press and massage for a count of 10. Release. Repeat for a total of 3 times.

5. Place middle fingers on the temples by coming out from the end of the eyebrows and locating soft depressions on the sides of the head (point E). Press and massage for a count of 10. Release. Repeat for a total of 3 times.

6. Palming. Rub hands together briskly until they are quite warm. Cup the hands over both eyes, fingers slightly crossed, right over left. Do not press the eyes. Hold for a count of 10. Then repeat for a total of 3 times, always feeling the warmth entering into the eyes from the hands.

7. Then rub eyes lightly with three middle fingers. Rub the bones around the eyes in a circular motion, starting from the inside corner of each eye next to the nose. Rub up the bridge of the nose, across the eyebrows, towards the temples, down and back around the lower rims of the eye sockets to the nose again. Do this 10 times. Pause. Repeat for a total of 3 cycles.

NOTE A: Rubbing in the opposite direction will weaken the eye muscles and cause wrinkles to appear. Always use a natural, healing cream as a lubricant.

NOTE B: For cataract or glaucoma, practice the first seven eye exercises up to 20 minutes daily. Whenever your eyes are tired, do the Eye Exercises, as they will completely revitalize your entire body in minutes. It is also good to do them in conjunction with exercises which strengthen the liver.

NOTE C: Once you have located the painful points, it is not necessary to continue pressing hard on these points. When you are doing the Eye

Exercises, even a very light touching of the points will accomplish the purpose of the exercise, which is to restore normal vision.
NOTE D: Use the first two points (A and B) for diagnosis. If it is painful at all when you press in deeply, then there is something wrong with the eyes and/or body. If it is puffy or dark under point B, water retention or lack of proper rest is indicated.

One may also practice additional exercises which will strengthen the eyes and the muscles surrounding them.

1. Begin by keeping the head straight, but with the eyes first looking up toward the ceiling and then down at the floor. Repeat this motion several times. The eyes should always move slowly and with deliberation.

2. Next, look to either side of the head.

3. Then look up and down into the opposite corners of the eyes.

4. Then rotate the eyes first in a clockwise direction, then in a counterclockwise direction. This will take about ten minutes to perform when done slowly.

5. Always follow these eye movements with a rubbing of the hands and a pressing of the palms onto the eyes to bring heat and energy into them.

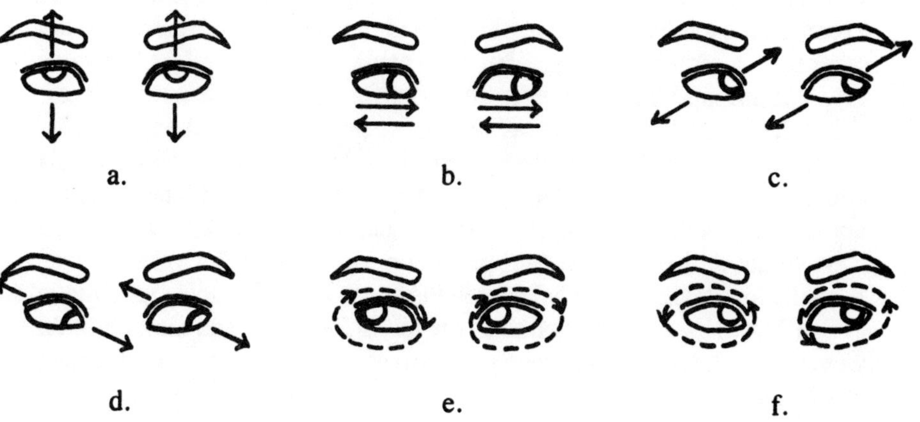

Figures 56a.—56f. Eye Motions.

If you practice these exercises consistently over a period of time, you may never need glasses to see clearly.

A student of mine and his family benefited greatly from the Eye Exercises. His problems first began after he left his job in the computer department of a San Francisco telephone company for a better job in San Jose. Because he was working as a trainee on three months probation at the San Jose company, his wife—then working as a nurse in a San Francisco hospital—could not leave her job and move away from San Francisco. Plus their house and four children were in San Francisco. So even if he was tired after hours of heavy concentration and computer training, he still had to drive for a total of 3 hours to and from work and fight traffic. When he did get home, he was overwhelmed by the demands of his four children. Not being able to stand the noise any longer, he retreated to his bedroom, locked the door, and collapsed on the bed. It was not long before his miserable outlook on life, lack of appetite for his wife's cooking, and indifference toward family and marital matters started explosive fights between him and his equally strained wife. Soon they agreed to a divorce. But before they took any legal action, they came to my office seeking advice. After carefully listening to both husband and wife, I discovered that they still loved each other and that the only things tearing them apart were the stress and tension of overwork. I therefore asked them to delay taking any legal action for two weeks, enough time to let the Eye Exercises take effect. I gave the husband the instructions for the exercises and asked him to do them when he drove on the emptier and safer sections of Highway 280. He could exercise both eyes by steering with the right hand as he exercised his left eye with his left hand and then switching hands to do the other eye. A month or so later they both came back to my office bearing a gift. The husband said the Eye Exercises performed a miracle on their lives. When he exercised his eyes as he drove, he was never tired when he reached home—he felt completely refreshed. He was able to play with his children, answer their questions, even help them do their homework; his appetite returned; he was able to fulfill his marital duties; and he was able to concentrate on his job and pass probation smoothly. Afterward, he was formally hired, and he was able to sell the house in San Francisco and move to San Jose. His wife also found a new job in San Jose, and their children were happy. They said they were starting a new life with more love for each other than ever before.

THE NOSE EXERCISE

The nose is the opening to the lungs. Symptoms such as allergies, runny nose, and blocked sinuses are the manifestations of weakness within the lungs. To strengthen the lungs, one should perform the Crane Exercise, which directs a flow of energy that helps restore any degenerative conditions within the pulmonary system. We can also help keep the lungs strong, as well as keep the sinuses healthy, by stimulating certain points around the nose. These are spots which open up into the meridians that supply the nose and surrounding areas with energy. By pressing these points, we insure a continual flow of energy through the nasal and sinus passages.

The exercise can be done several times throughout the day, as many times as necessary to help correct sinus or nasal problems. But if time does not allow it, doing the exercise once, after the Eye Exercise, with the aid of a healing herbal cream will suffice.

1. Using the tip of the index or the second fingers of each hand, press down with heavy pressure on the three points as described below.

2. Begin at the base of the nose and press these points for about ten seconds. Then rub these points briefly.

3. Next, press the points midway up on either side of the nose for about ten seconds. Then rub briefly.

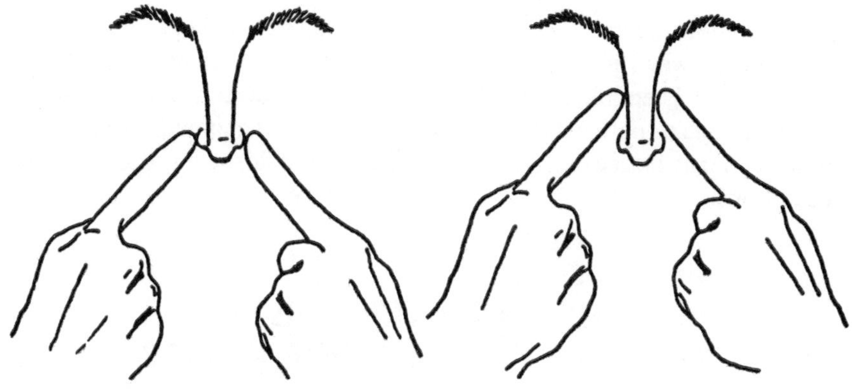

a. b.

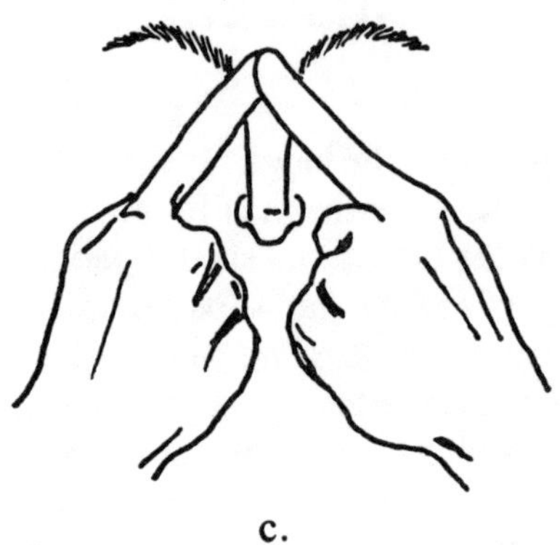

c.

Figures 57a—57c. Nose Exercise.

4. Press the point midway between the eyebrows (the third eye) with both fingers. Then rub briefly.

5. Repeat this progression three times, always beginning with the lower points and ending by pressing the point corresponding to the third eye.

6. Rub in a continual flowing motion, starting at the lowest point, passing through the second and third points, then continuing up through the middle of the forehead. Repeat this movement for a total of three times.

Throughout the exercise, the pressure exerted should be penetrating and deep. Often when just beginning, the points will be sensitive or slightly painful. This is an indication of weakness or blockages within the meridian. Continue to perform this exercise daily and the pain will disappear in time. You may notice that you will acquire fewer colds, allergies, and sinus conditions.

THE EAR EXERCISE OR "BEATING THE HEAVENLY DRUM"

Whether it be daytime or nighttime, one's environment never rests.

When you are sleeping you may think you hear nothing, but the ears are still receiving stimuli. Taoist teachings show a way to rest the ears. They call this exercise "Beating the Heavenly Drum".

This exercise stimulates and gives rest to the inner ear. It is very important to keep your ears healthy, and by following this exercise you will insure good hearing into old age. Many diseases of the ears, such as ringing and partial deafness, can be helped or cured by using this exercise.

In Chinese medicine, the ears are regarded as the opening to the kidneys. So if you do have problems with your ears, it is a warning signal that you have a weakness in your kidneys. It is important then to also practice the Kidney Exercise along with the Ear Exercise.

The ears lie in line with, and are connected to, the pineal gland, which, as you may recall, is the center for spiritual awareness. Practicing the Ear Exercise stimulates the pineal gland and helps to keep it healthy and energized. You may find you feel very tranquil after performing this exercise.

Practice the Ear Exercise in the morning after working on the nose. Then you may perform it as often as you like during the day. Those who suffer from ear problems may want to practice this exercise many times during the day until the condition improves.

1. Place the index fingers of each hand on the outside of the ears and fold over the outside flaps of skin which lie next to the opening of the inner ear canal, so that you seal off the ear from the outside.

2. Using the tips of your second fingers, tap gently on the fingernails of your index fingers. When done properly, you will hear a metallic sound much like the beating of a drum. Tap a regular rhythm, slowly, twelve to thirty-six times.

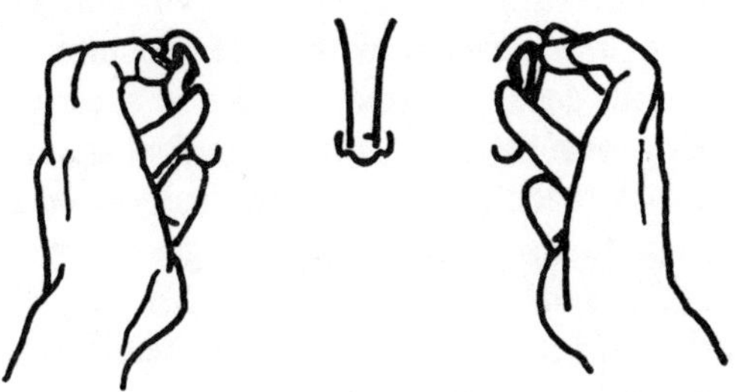

Figure 58. Ear Exercise (Beating the Heavenly Drum).

3. Pause. Then repeat for a total of three times.

NOTE A: When you first close off your ears, before you begin tapping, you will hear a sound much like that made by a waterfall. The ear is still working. After following this exercise for a few days, the sound of the waterfall will cease and will be replaced by a calm silence.

MOUTH EXERCISES

In addition to the other areas of the face, we need to stimulate as well the mouth, teeth and gums to keep them healthy and strong. We continually use our mouths for talking, eating, and kissing. So in order to keep this area strong and prevent tooth decay and gum problems like gingivitis, the Mouth Exercises should be practiced.

The Tongue and Saliva Exercise

The tongue is recognized as the opening to the heart. Feelings of hate, love, sympathy, and anger reside in the heart and are stimulated by the tongue. When the tongue is used in kissing, passion rises from the heart.

Saliva, or "Heavenly Water", is sacred to the Taoists and is treated with respect for the power it holds as a natural healing water. It helps to kill germs in the mouth and may be used as a form of medicine. It may also be used to treat infections. If you cut yourself and there are no other healing aids available, put the cut in your mouth or spread some of your saliva over it. The saliva will help clean it out and destroy germs that might otherwise lead to infection. Interestingly, it is now known that saliva triggers the production of a particular hormone within the structure of the teeth which helps to prevent tooth decay. Further, saliva is a very important aid in digestion, and along with the teeth, forms the first step in breaking down foodstuffs before they reach the stomach. So saliva that is evenly distributed between food particles will increase the digestive system's capacity to absorb nutrients. (You can benefit from this property by chewing your food until it is in liquid form.) Because saliva is so valuable to human existence, the glands that produce it must be protected.

To keep the heart healthy and insure the continuing strength of the salivary glands into old age, Taoists devised the Tongue and Saliva Exercise. The literal English translation of this exercise is: "The Red Dragon dances over the ocean to make the wind, rain and clouds." (The Red Dragon is the tongue and the ocean is the saliva.) This one sentence captures the exercise's ability to wash out and clean the mouth and teeth and stimulate the heart.

This exercise may be done after meals, upon waking to remove bad breath, and at other appropriate times.

1. Roll your tongue around the inside of your mouth and across your gums and teeth. Use your tongue as you would a toothbrush.

2. As you roll your tongue around your mouth, saliva will be secreted by the salivary glands. Do not swallow it, but allow it to collect until you have a mouthful of saliva.

3. Swish the saliva around as if you were using a mouthwash. Wash the entire inside of your mouth including the gums and in between the teeth.

4. Divide the saliva into three equal parts and swallow each part separately and slowly until your mouth is clear. As you swallow it, feel it descend to your stomach. You may begin to feel the energy which the "Heavenly Water" brings to your stomach.

Gum Pressure Exercise

There are also points at the top and bottom of the lips which may be pressed to stimulate the meridians that supply energy to the mouth, teeth and gums. This exercise may be done in the mornings, after meals, or whenever appropriate.

1. Press the points designated in figure 59. Press with a firm and steady pressure and follow with a rubbing movement to energize this area. Repeat three times.

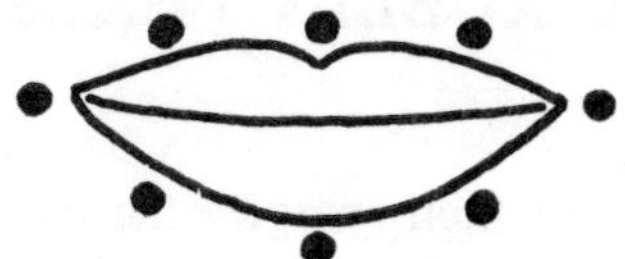

Figure 59. Gum Pressure Exercise.

Teeth Clicking Exercise

The teeth are vital parts of the digestive system. They break up food and distribute saliva throughout the food particles. One needs to protect the teeth from decaying, because if one cannot chew properly, one will not be able to digest food properly. The resultant decreased capacity to absorb the nutritive elements from food develops into a generally weakened internal system. To protect the teeth, one needs to do the Teeth Clicking Exercise.

Also, the body tends to loosen up and become vulnerable to outside germs during sexual intercourse, orgasm, and while moving the bowels. Teeth clicking or teeth clenching during these moments helps protect the body and keep up one's natural defenses.

A sign of old age is often loose teeth as well as loose joints. Clicking the teeth, as well as clenching the teeth during the day, will help tighten the joints of the body and keep the teeth healthy.

When practiced in the morning, this exercise will help awaken you. When practiced during the day, it will help to keep your mind alert.

1. Click the teeth together thirty-six times. This strengthens the teeth and gums.

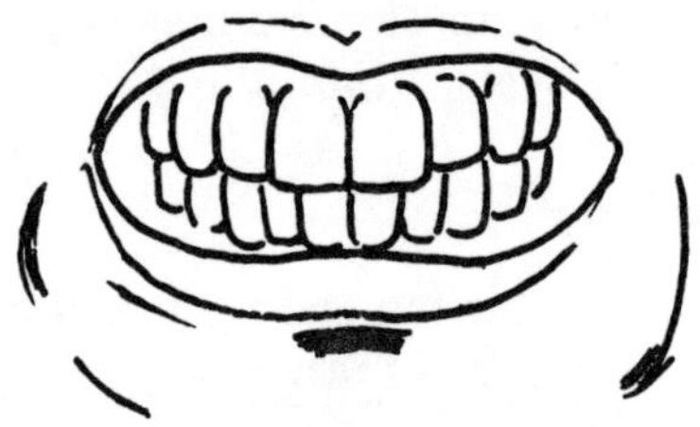

Figure 60. Teeth Clicking Exercise.

FACE RUBBING EXERCISE

After all the exercises which energize the individual parts of the face have been practiced, you need to stimulate the skin and facial muscles:

1. Rub your hands together vigorously.

2. Press your palms against your face so that you feel the warmth in your hands enter the skin and penetrate into the muscles. Feel the energy being absorbed by the cells throughout your face.

3. Rub your hands in outward circular motions around your face. Work your fingers and hands up through the bridge of your nose, through your third eye, and out across your forehead, continuing down your temples and cheeks and across your chin and mouth, then crossing back up along your nose. Continue rubbing for as long as you wish.

NOTE: You may want to stop occasionally to rub your hands together to bring more heat and energy into your face. Practice this exercise whenever your facial muscles become tired. This will help to reduce the formation of wrinkles and bring a glow to your complexion.

THYROID EXERCISE

The thyroid gland controls our bodies' metabolism. By massaging the thyroid area, energy will be sent into the thyroid to help it function more normally. Thus metabolism will be helped, enabling the body to eliminate more poisons and toxins. Digestion and absorption of nutrients will also improve. And thyroid medicine or iodine—both dangerous to take—will become unnecessary.

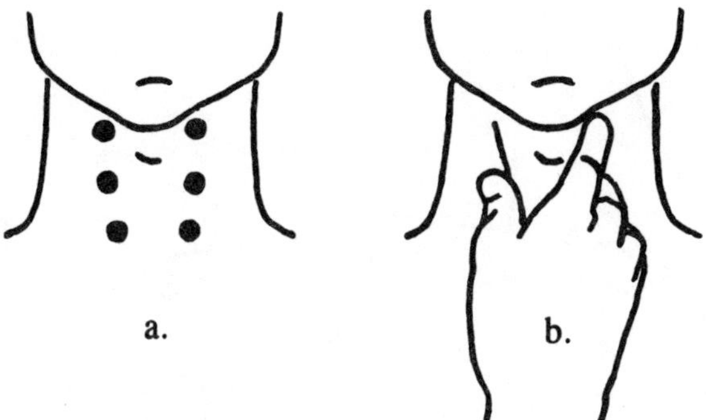

Figures 61a and 61b. Thyroid Exercise.

TECHNIQUES FOR RELIEVING PAIN

This simple exercise helps relieve upper back, shoulder or neck pain and may be practiced whenever discomfort is felt in the upper spine. Using this exercise can eliminate the need for aspirin.

1. Assume the sitting position.

2. If pain is felt in the upper right quadrant of the back, allow your right arm to lie motionless on your thighs. If the pain is on the left, do the same with your left arm.

3. Extend your left arm out in front of your chest with the fingers pointed.

4. Fix your eyes on the fingers of your left hand and slowly begin to move your left hand up and out to your left side. Keep your breathing normal, and raise your arm as high as possible.

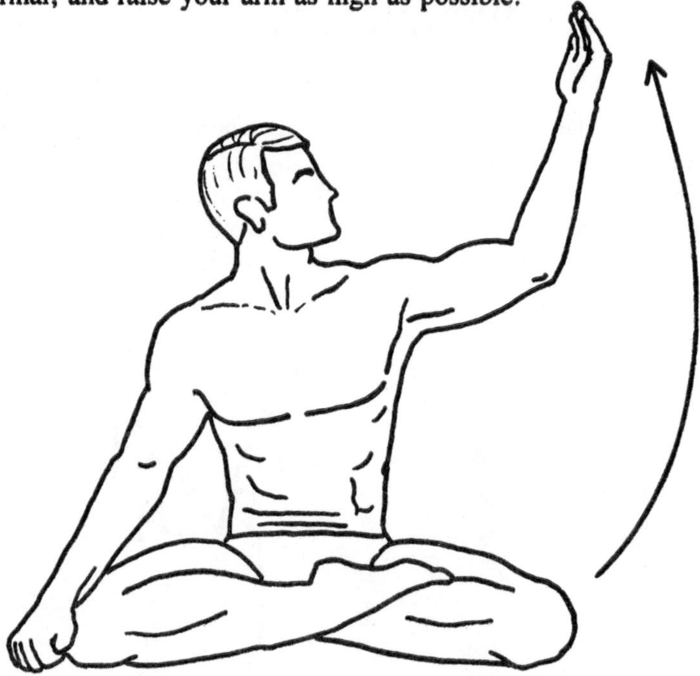

Figure 62. Pain Relief Exercise.

5. Slowly lift your arm to its original position.

6. Repeat the movement for a total of 7 times.

NOTE: This exercise helps to lure the attention away from pain in the upper trunk and bring healing energy into the sore area. Throughout the exercise, keep your attention focused on the hand that is being raised. If your mind wanders, bring it back to your hand. You may wish to synchronize your breathing with the hand raising. In that case inhale as the arm moves upward and exhale as you bring the arm down.

HANDS, ARMS, AND UPPER BODY EXERCISES

These exercises are similar to those practiced in T'ai Chi Chuan, Kung Fu, and Karate. The exercises build up the strength of the arms and hands, tone the muscles and nerves of the arms, increase the circulation of the blood, and energize the heart, lung, and Heart Constrictor meridians which lie along the arm.

The secret of these exercises is that they increase the energy within the arm, not just the bulk of muscles. By concentrating on the flow of energy within the arms and hands, your arms will grow strong and will therefore tire less when you are performing manual tasks. The exercises help heal all problems of the arms, including arthritis, bursitis, and tennis elbow.

Arm and Hand Pressing Exercise

This exercise may be practiced sitting, standing, or lying down.

1. Place your right hand in close to your right armpit with your palm facing front.

2. Slowly move your hand away from your chest and extend it straight out, leading with the heel of the hand. Keeping your fingers relaxed and breathing normally, try to feel that you are pushing the air away from your body.

3. Repeat this movement for a total of 7 times.

4. Repeat the movement 7 times again with the left hand.

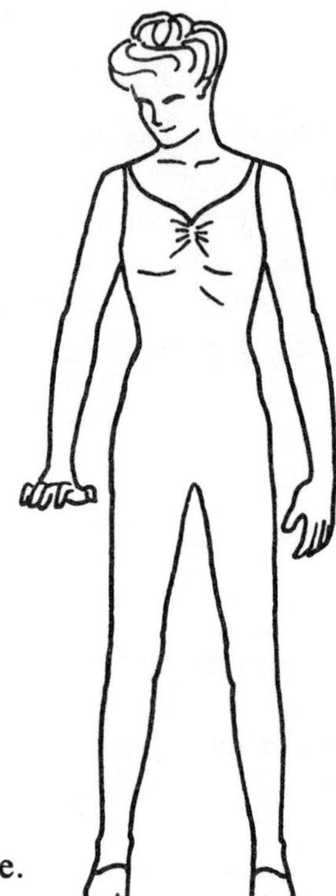

Figure 63.
Arm and Hand Pressing Exercise.

NOTE: When practicing the Arm and Hand Pressing Exercise, never force the movements. Use little pressure and feel that your hands are firm but soft and warm and full of energy. Always concentrate fully on what you are doing, otherwise you will not be able to stimulate the energy so that it flows properly through the arm, wrist, and hand.

Hand and Arm Exercise

This exercise, like the previous one, is used to energize and strengthen the arms and hands. This is a subtle but very dynamic exercise which may be easily overlooked, but which, when practiced, brings many beneficial results. This exercise also helps heal problems associated with the shoulder, arms and hands, and works to kill the pain accompanying such problems as tennis elbow, bursitis, and arthritis. Practice this exercise when you have pain in any part of the upper limbs, and continue the treatment until you have regained the complete mobility of the injured part.

1. Lie down on the floor on your stomach and place your palms on the floor shoulder-width apart and slightly in front of each shoulder. The forearms and elbows should remain on the floor throughout the exercise. Keep your chest and head up off the floor and breathe normally. Allow your legs to relax and keep a light but steady pressure on your arms.

2. Hold this position for several seconds with a deep and concentrated attention.

3. Relax your mind and turn you head back to look at the heel of your right foot. As you inhale, feel the air come in through that foot, travel up the leg and through your body so that it comes into your right arm and down to your fingers.

4. As you exhale, send the air back out of your arm and down the right leg so that it leaves your body through the right foot.

5. Turn your head the other way and repeat the breathing using your left foot, leg, and arm to follow the air through your body.

6. Repeat the total exercise 7 times each time you practice it.

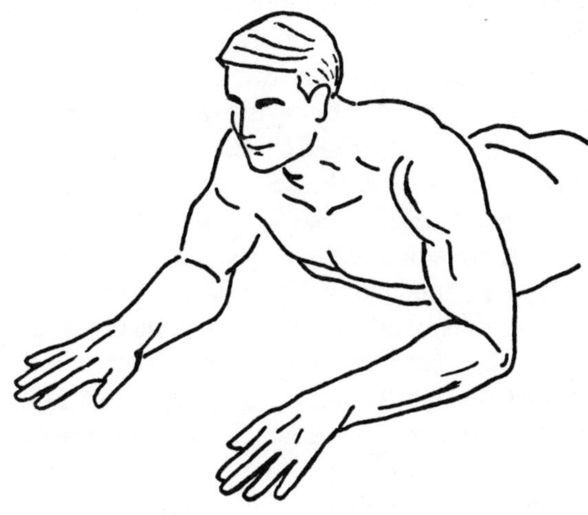

Figure 64. Hand and Arm Exercise.

NOTE A: For the exercise to be effective, you must concentrate deeply for the duration of the exercise. If you find that your mind wanders during the process, then begin again. At first you will not be able to detect the flow of energy through your body, but with practice you will come to feel the energy as it enters your foot, travels up your leg, and enters into your arm and hands. The in-flow of energy will help to heal any injury or disease you may have in your arms or shoulders.

Through the use of the breathing and deep concentration techniques, you will be stimulating the energy meridians along the legs and arms that supply energy to the upper limbs. By practicing this exercise you will not only be increasing the flow of energy to the upper body, but you will also be increasing the circulation of blood as well.

THE LUNG EXERCISE

This exercise helps heal any kind of lung problem, even a common cold. It strengthens the entire breathing system, including the skin, which is often called the "third lung".

Exercising the lungs is vitally important to our health. Full expansion and contraction of the lungs allow for full absorption of energy and help the lungs combat disease-causing agents. (Babies are born with this knowledge for they exercise their lungs often by crying. But when these babies learn to hold their emotions in to try to remain calm, pressures begin to build inside. This could be the basis for the phrase "the good die young", since the "good" control their feelings and reactions. On the other hand the "bad"—those who are emotionally undisciplined and release their emotions readily—live without internal pressure, and so they live longer.) When lungs are healthy they are more capable of handling the many disease-causing agents that they continuously filter out of the air. (The nose, although a wonderful filtering device, cannot filter out every microscopic particle in the air.) So cigarette smokers whose lungs are still healthy will cough a great deal. Coughing is a good sign, for it at least shows that the lungs are trying to rid themselves of toxins.

To determine the health of the lungs and body, one should measure the length of the inhalation and exhalation. If the exhalation is longer than the inhalation, ill health is indicated, since more is going out than is coming in. If the inhalation is longer, that is a healthy sign, since more energy is taken in.

Snoring is an example of improper breathing brought about by incorrect sleeping positions. Correct sleeping positions are those that encourage nasal breathing.

It is even more important that asthma sufferers breathe through the nose. Besides being an air filter, the nose also warms the air to body temperature before it hits the delicate lung tissues. If the air temperature is too cold, the bronchial tubes are stimulated, and asthma can result. The bronchial tubes are tubular structures which make up the greater portion of the lungs and which have hair-like projections (cilia) pointing straight within. When mucous or cold air flattens the cilia, the bronchial tubes constrict, blocking the passage of air into the lungs. Then asthma results. So joggers, walkers, and soldiers who are trained in the cold, early mornings are likelier to develop asthma. Asthma sufferers should protect themselves thoroughly from the cold air by wearing a mask when it is absolutely necessary to go out in the cold. They should also help the cilia heal by nourishing them with herbs especially formulated to help that area. (Regular foods will not help.) And they should do the Lung Exercise.

1. Stand with your feet shoulder-width apart and parallel to each other. Your back should be straight, your chin slightly toward your chest, and your head erect, as if the back of your neck is stretching upward.

2. Exhale all the air from your lungs and clasp your hands behind your back.

3. Now inhale slowly, expanding your lungs and pushing your hands away from your back. Keep your chin tucked into your chest, and use only your chest to breathe with while practicing this exercise.

4. Exhaling, drop your hands and bring your arms out in front of you. Continue to raise your arms, bringing your hands up toward your head and then around behind your back and back up in front of your body, completing one cycle. Your fingers should be pointed throughout the rotation.

5. Interlace your fingers behind your back and begin the exercise again on the inhalation.

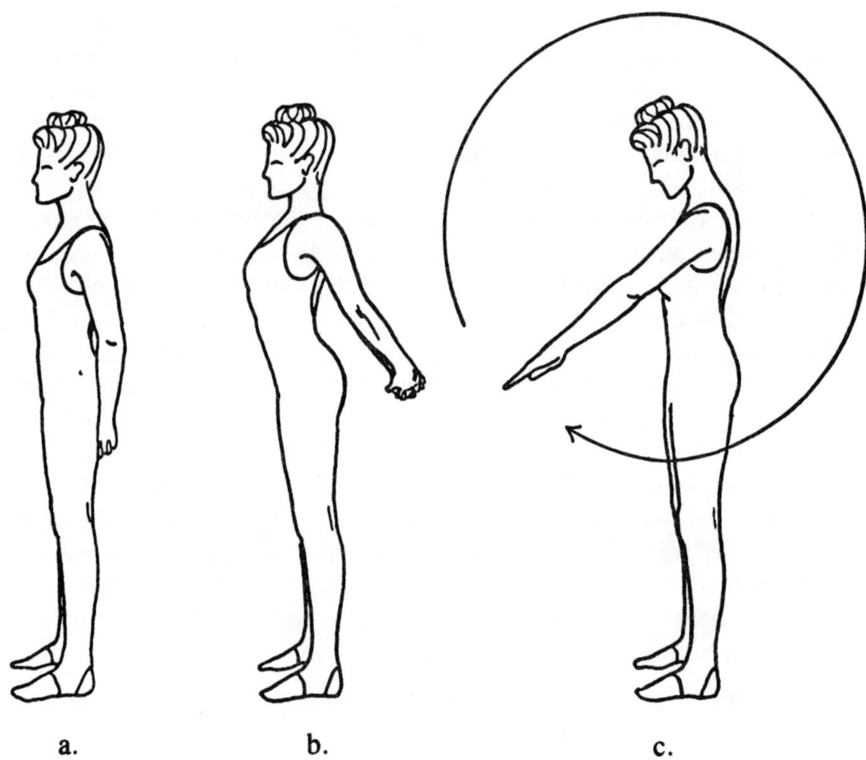

Figures 65a — 65c. Lung Exercise.

6. Repeat for a total of 7 times.

NOTE: As you inhale air into your lungs, feel the fresh energy come in to invigorate the lung tissues. As you exhale, feel all the germs, stale air, and toxins leave your lungs.

THE HEART EXERCISES

The following exercises heal and prevent diseases and problems of the heart, to keep the heart strong and healthy. We need to pay particular attention to the heart, because it is an organ that works constantly from its appearance in the womb to the moment its owner dies; there is no rest for the heart.

Beside these exercises, Taoism also provides methods for helping a heart-attack victim. In case of a real heart attack, rub and pinch the fifth, or smallest, finger. The endings of the heart meridian can be found there. If the heart really stops, use the fingers to pinch a point above the middle of the upper lip. Place the forefinger between the upper lip and teeth and the thumb outside the upper lip, and pinch the flesh with these fingers. Pinch

Figure 66. Pressure Point on Upper Lip.

very hard. Doing so has revived even those who have died from heart attacks. Several nurses have told me that they actually brought several dead patients—they were pronounced dead by the doctors—back to life by using this technique. The whole hospital buzzed with excitement—everyone thought it was a miracle. Unfortunately, the doctors did not believe it.

Heart Energizing Exercise

This exercise strengthens the heart tissue and surrounding blood vessels.

1. Sit or stand in a comfortable position with your hands extended out in front of your chest at the level of the shoulders. The finger tips of each hand should almost come together, but keep a little distance between them.

2. Keep your eyes focused on the tips of the fingers, or close them gently.

3. Next, see if you can feel a current of energy flow between your fingers, from one hand to the other.

4. Hold your arms out in front of you for as long as you comfortably can, and keep your concentration on the energy flow.

5. Let your arms relax for a few minutes, then repeat for a total of 3 times.

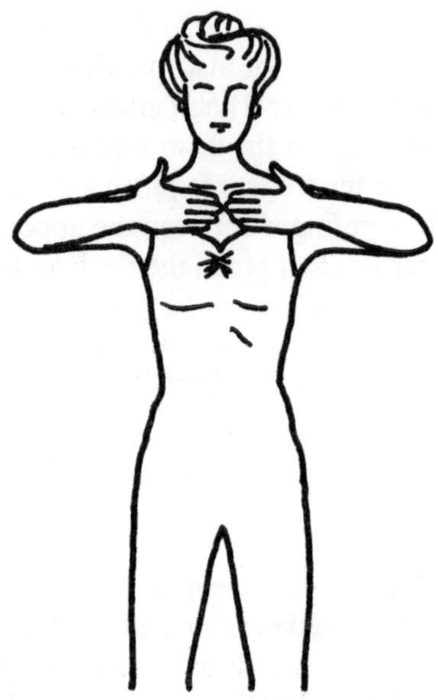

Figure 67. Heart Energizing Exercise.

This exercise creates a flow of energy which comes in through the fingers of the right hand, comes across the chest and into the heart, then passes out through the left arm, hand, and fingers. As the energy passes through the heart, it strengthens the heart tissue and surrounding blood vessels. If at first you are unable to perceive this energy flow, develop your patience and keep practicing the exercise. You will quickly begin to perceive a tingling sensation in the fingertips. With practice, you will be able to feel the entire circle of energy as it passes through your arms, body, and heart. Then you will know that you are building a stronger heart.

Strengthening the Nerves Leading to the Heart

Please refer the first pose of the Twelve Nerve Exercises.

Heart Healing Exercise

This exercise clears the brain and heart of disease-causing agents by helping the practitioner relax and reduce the stress on the heart. It can also remove diseases and problems of the heart.

The heart exercise may be practiced morning, noon and night, depending upon the seriousness of the problem. If you have a weak heart, practice it once a day. If there are palpitations of the heart or angina, practice it at least twice a day. If you have had a heart attack, then this exercise needs to be performed at least three times a day. The exercise may also be practiced as preventative medicine to keep a strong heart healthy.

1. Lie down on on a firm surface so that only the left side of your body is touching the surface. This exercise may only be practiced lying on the left side.

2. Extend your left arm so that it lies straight along the left side of your body with your hand down toward your left knee. Your left arm will press firmly into your chest and heart region as your body lies on top of it. Your left leg should be straight, and the right knee should be bent slightly. Your right arm will lie gently down on the floor in front of your body with your hand a little bit above your head. Allow your head and face to relax on the floor. Your left arm should exert quite a bit of pressure on your heart so that during the exercise the heart remains constricted. This prevents the heart from overreacting.

3. Close your eyes and slowly exhale all the air from your lungs. As the air leaves your body, feel the disease, weakness, and pain leave your heart.

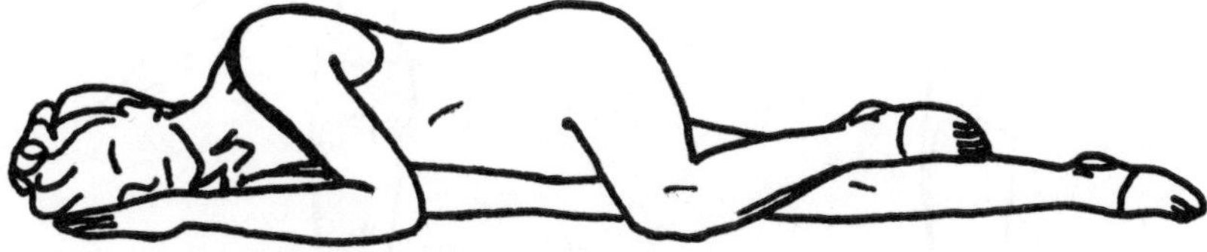

Figure 68. Strengthening the Nerves Leading to the Heart.

4. As you slowly inhale, feel the fresh, clean energy enter your heart, and feel the heart become strong and revitalized.

NOTE A: As you inhale, you may imagine that a mist or warm steam is coming into your heart and penetrating every crevice within your heart. As you exhale, feel the weakness and disease go out of your heart with the steam. You want to wash out the heart. At all times the inhalation and exhalation should be very slow and done only through the nose.

NOTE B: For this exercise to be effective, you must concentrate with all the power of your mind. If you find that your mind has wandered during the exercise, begin again.

ABDOMINAL STRENGTHENING EXERCISE

This exercise strengthens the intestines, colon, and internal organs in the abdomen. It tightens the muscles of the abdomen, and corrects such problems as constipation and diarrhea. It also adjusts the posture and strengthens the spine.

1. Stand with your arms stretched out in front of your body and held slightly above chest level.

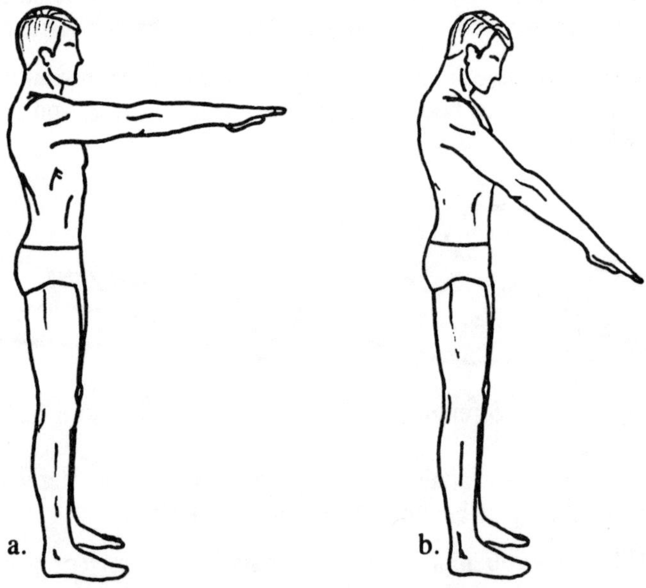

Figures 69a and 69b. Abdominal Strengthening Exercise.

2. Inhale completely, so that your lungs fill with air and your chest expands.

3. Exhale slowly, using only your abdominal muscles to force the air out of your lungs. As you exhale, slowly drop your arms down to your sides and tighten the abdominal muscles as much as possible.

4. Then bring your arms in front of you again and begin the next inhalation.

5. Repeat for a total of 7 times.

WEIGHT REDUCTION EXERCISE

As you may already know, being excessively overweight can be dangerous to your health. This does not mean that it is wrong to be overweight, but merely that it goes against the natural laws of healing.

Blood which is normally sent to the head and brain remains in the abdominal cavity to aid the digestive organs with their increased work load. The heart must work harder (and because of this excess strain, becomes critically weakened and more likely to collapse) due to the increase of fatty tissues and, usually, because of the weakened circulation in the arteries and veins. As a result of fats and lipids in the blood, high blood pressure results. Excessive weight also brings on physical as well as mental fatigue and sluggishness by overworking the system. There is usually accompanying lower back pain because of the increased load on the spine. It is said that when your abdomen is larger than your chest, you can buy a box to prepare for your funeral.

The Weight Reduction Exercise helps bring down the weight to a manageable level and helps adjust the back to keep it healthy and strong.

When practicing this exercise, remember never to force or push yourself beyond your limits. Acquire patience and steadiness in your practice.

Part One

1. Stand against a wall so that your heels, buttocks, upper back, and head are against the wall.

2. Inhaling through your nose, stretch your body upward, pulling

your abdomen in as far as possible so your chest expands fully. Keep your arms by your sides. Your shoulders should feel as if they are expanding and pressing against the wall.

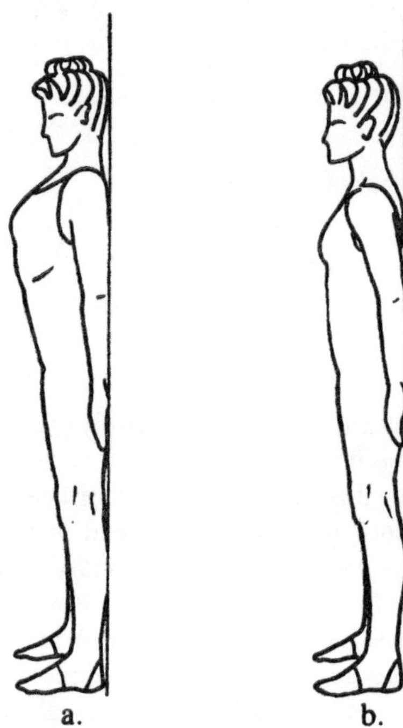

Figures 70a and 70b. Part I.

3. Exhale as quickly as possible through your mouth. Blow the breath out fully and push your abdomen outward. Your entire body will tighten automatically on the exhale if done properly.

4. Practice this inhale-exhale repetition 7 to 12 times.

You will find that with consistent practice, the muscles in your abdomen and belly will tighten and become toned and strengthened. Excess fat, water, and flesh will be eliminated, and the belly will shrink.

Part Two

1. Stand away from the wall and bring your heels off the floor so that

you will be standing as high on your toes as possible.

2. Keeping your spine erect and straight, bend your knees slightly as if you were going to sit on a chair. Your arms will fall at a 45 degree angle from your body.

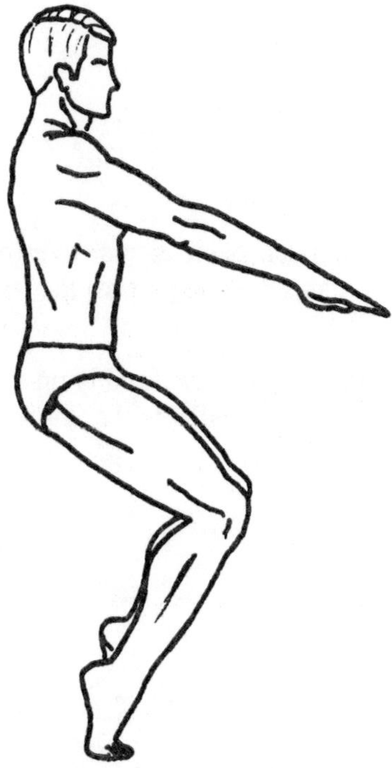

Figure 71. Part II.

3. Keeping your breath regular, stay in this position from 10 to 20 seconds, or longer if possible.

NOTE: At first it will be impossible to keep your back straight and your heels up very far. With practice and practice, you will be able to get your heels perpendicular to the floor, your thighs parallel to the floor, and your back straight.

This pose strengthens and tones the thighs, calves and ankles. It makes the abdominal muscles strong and increases the circulation in the legs and body, as well as strengthening the back and the nerves in the body. It also stimulates the meridians of the bladder, gallbladder, and stomach. These meridians lie along the legs, and so it helps to reduce water retention and excessive weight and lowers the blood pressure.

Always practice both parts of the exercise at the same sitting as they balance and complement each other.

STOMACH HEALING EXERCISE

This exercise helps stomach pain, ulcers, over-acidity, flatulence, indigestion, and stomach cancer. It helps take the focus of the mind away from the stomach.

1. Sit in a comfortable position, preferably on a chair with your feet flat on the floor, your thighs parallel to the floor, and your spine erect and straight.

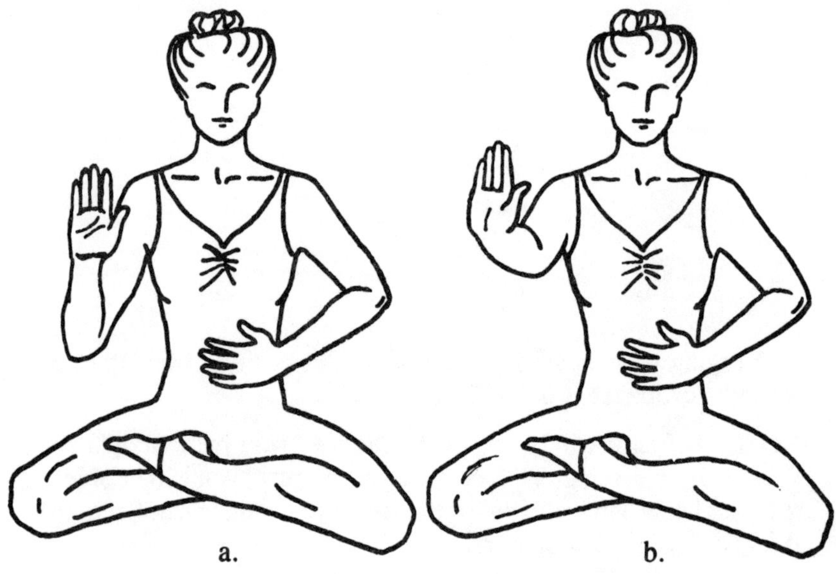

Figures 72a and 72b. Stomach Healing Exercise.

2. Place your left palm on the stomach area slightly to the left of the abdominal cavity.

3. Inhaling, slowly move the palm of your right hand away from your chest, concentrating and fixing your eyes on the tip of the fingers. As you push your hand and arm forward, feel that you're pushing a heavy object with the heel of your hand. Your eyes should intently follow the movements of your right hand throughout this exercise.

4. Exhaling, slowly bring your right hand back to your chest.

5. Perform this in and out movement for a total of 7 times.

NOTE: As you move your hand away from your chest, feel a band of energy moving out of your stomach. The right hand is draining the energy. Then feel the left hand absorb new energy into the stomach. For this exercise to be effective, you must concentrate deeply on what you are doing. The exercise should be done slowly, with total synchronization of your breath, mind, and hand movements.

THE LIVER EXERCISE

Besides the lungs, there are two other main filters of the body: the kidneys and liver. The liver filters toxins from the body; therefore, we must perform the Liver Exercise to keep the liver functioning properly.

Throughout this exercise, as with all the exercises, you want to keep your mind on what you are doing. It helps if you can feel the flow of energy across your chest. Keeping your mind on the task helps to increase the benefits derived from doing the exercise as well as serving to unify your mind with your body. Practice this exercise in the morning after you have performed the Kidney Exercise.

1. Sit or lie down in a comfortable position. (Refer to the descriptions of the proper way to sit and lie down.)

2. Place the palm of your right hand on the right lateral side of your body so that it lies at the base of your rib cage.

3. Push your hand across the front of your chest following the line made by the lower rib bones of your chest. Rub up toward your

sternum and then down toward the left lateral side of your chest.

4. Rubbing once from the right to the left constitutes one turn. Repeat the movement for a total of 36 times.

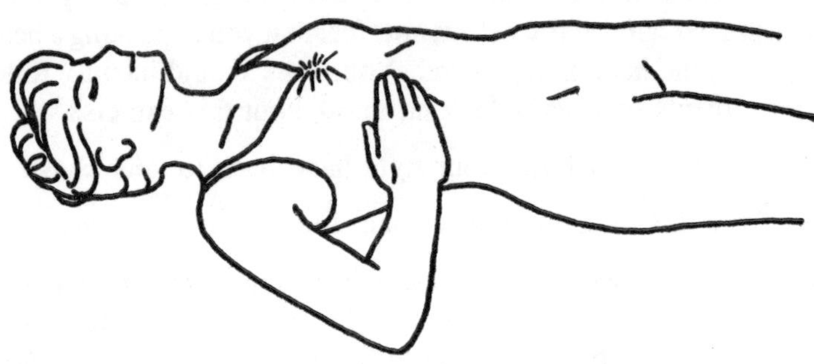

Figure 73. Liver Exercise.

NOTE A: The heel of your hand should exert pressure on the skin as you rub your hand across it. The liver lies just below the skin under the right rib cage on the right side of the body. The pressure exerted by the hand rubbing across the chest stimulates the flow of energy as well as the circulation of blood to the liver.

NOTE B: You may also use your left hand to rub across your chest, beginning at the left lateral side and again following the outline made by the lower ribs as you rub across your chest to the right side. The stomach lies just below the skin on the left side of the chest, and so this hand rubbing keeps the energy flowing to the stomach.

Do this exercise 36 times also. You may want to alternate hands, starting first with the right hand for one turn, then using your left hand for one turn, continuing the rotation until you have performed 36 rubbings with each hand.

Practicing both forms of this exercise helps build up the relationship between the digestive organs, stomach, and liver. One wants to push the energy from one organ to the other so that the two organs will work together smoothly.

Recently, while on a lecture tour, I had reason to demonstrate this exercise. I asked my audience to perform it for themselves. I noted at the time one woman who entered into the spirit of it with obvious gusto.

Several weeks later, that same woman telephoned my office to ask if she might fly up to see me. When she arrived, to my great astonishment, she said she had made the trip only to thank me. "For what?" I asked. "For the Liver Exercise," she replied. "I have had liver trouble all my life. When you demonstrated the Liver Exercise at your lecture, I said to myself, 'What have I got to lose?' and began doing the exercise. Two weeks later, at my regular checkup, my physician told me my liver condition had improved sixty percent, and he couldn't imagine why. So that's why I'm here. Simply to thank you!"

THE KIDNEY EXERCISE

This exercise stimulates the adrenal glands and the kidneys, which lie directly behind the small of the back. Lower back pain is often caused by a weakness in the kidneys. Two factors which help weaken the kidneys are drinking an excess of liquids and standing on the feet for prolonged periods. By practicing this exercise you will be strengthening, energizing, and healing the kidneys and adrenals. By association you will be helping lower back problems as well as strengthening the eyes, as the kidneys are also connected with the eyes. Further, the exercise helps keep the skin smooth and beautiful, as the kidneys' capacity for filtering toxins is kept at a maximum, and encourages strong sexual feelings by energizing the glandular system.

This exercise may by practiced in a standing or prone position.

1. Rub your hands together vigorously to get the energy flowing into your palms and fingers.

2. Place your palms on the small of your back. Keep your upper body tilted slightly forward. Feel the energy and heat flowing from your hands into your back and kidneys.

3. Massage the small of your back by rubbing up and down and then in a circular motion across your back.

4. Clench your fingers together to form two fists and hit the small of your back with the back of your hands. Pummel the area softly for a few seconds.

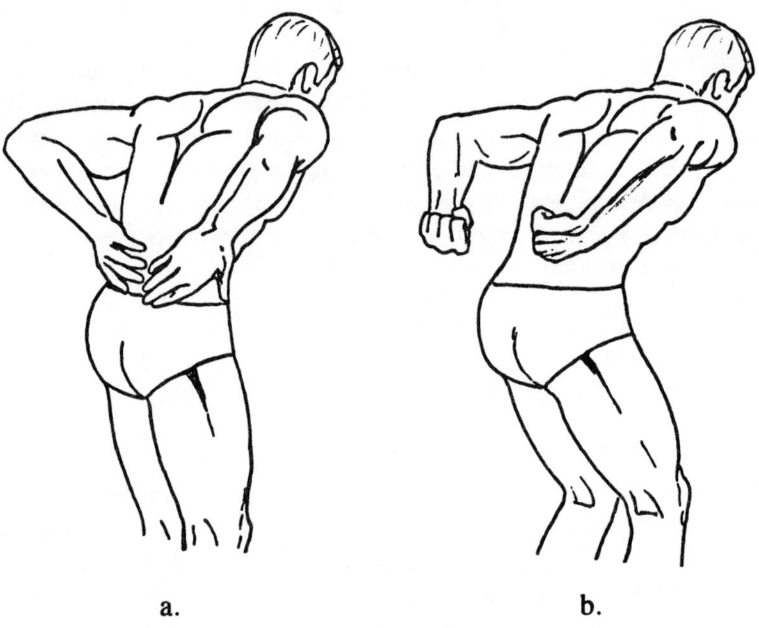

Figures 74a and 74b. Kidney Exercise.

5. Repeat the rubbing and pummeling action for a total of three times.

6. This exercise should be done in the morning or whenever there is lower back pain.

THE LOWER BACK EXERCISES

Pain itself is not a disease but rather a signal of an existing or developing problem. Lower back pain is no exception. Lumbago, lordosis, slipped discs, and other back problems limit movement and create unnecessary pain. The Lower Back Exercises are designed to strengthen the spine, the muscles around the abdomen, vertebrae, tail bone, and kidneys. When done daily, they can correct lower back problems.

Exercise 1

1. Sit in a comfortable position and bring your knees up to your chest. Hold around the knees with your hands. If possible, grab onto your elbows with your hands.

2. As you inhale, straighten your spine and lift your head upward.

3. As you exhale, hunch your back so your lower abdomen becomes like a ball—as if you were about to roll over backward. Your head will come forward toward your knees.

4. Repeat this straightening and hunching movement for a total of 7 times. Seven is the number of creation, and this exercise will help create a new back. Practice all the movements slowly, with your full concentration on your lower back.

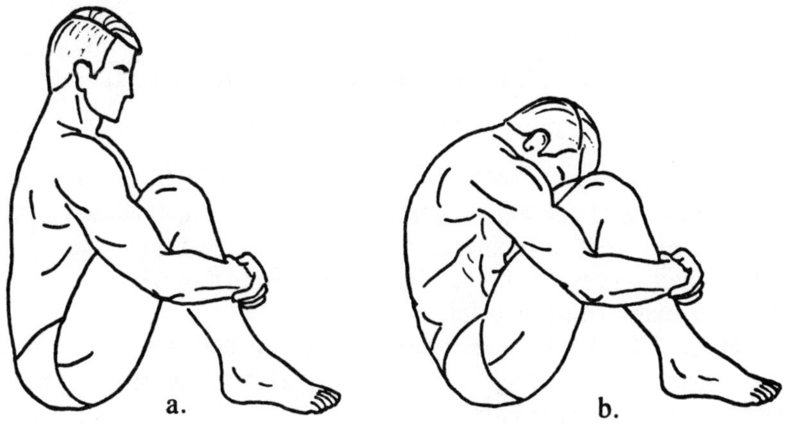

Figures 75a and 75b. Exercise1.

Exercise 2

This exercise may be done while lying on your back.

1. Place one hand under your lower back and feel the hollow space under your lower spine.

2. Tuck under your tail bone and drop your lower back to the floor as much as possible.

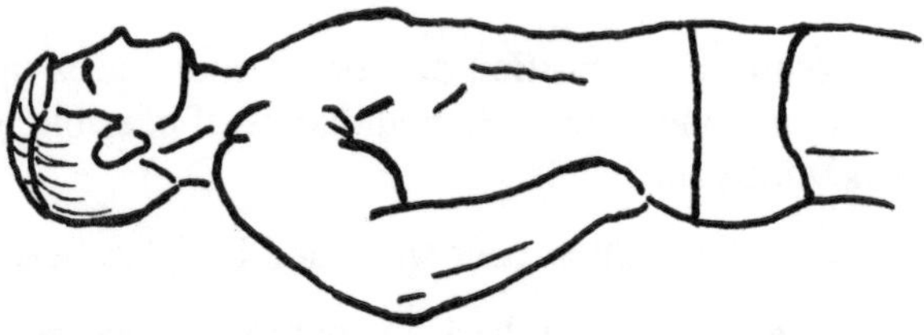

Figure 76. Exercise 2.

3. Release your back to the beginning position, and start again.

4. Repeat this progression for a total of 7 times, which completes one cycle.

THE SUN WORSHIP EXERCISE

Sunlight represents a positive, energizing force which we can harness to help cleanse our bodies as well as our minds. Sunlight enables the skin of our bodies to produce vitamin D, a necessary nutrient for good health. The combination of fresh air and sunlight has been used throughout the ages as a tonic for many ailments of the body.

The Sun Worship Exercise works to wash the body both on the outside and on the inside, cleaning out disease and germs, and restoring a feeling of vibrant and glowing health.

Normally we clean our mouth and teeth and the rest of the body when we wash, but we never really think to clean the rectum and anus thoroughly. This negligence can cause an accumulation of germs at the anal opening, causing weakness to occur and possibly hemorrhoids, polyps, or cancer of the colon or anus. Sunlight is an ever-present and free source of energy which we can bathe ourselves in to wash out all disease and weakness and restore our energy to its proper level.

1. Turn your body so that the spine faces the sun.

2. Lean over so that the sunlight is allowed to come into the anal opening. (This exercise needs to be done in a nude for best results.)

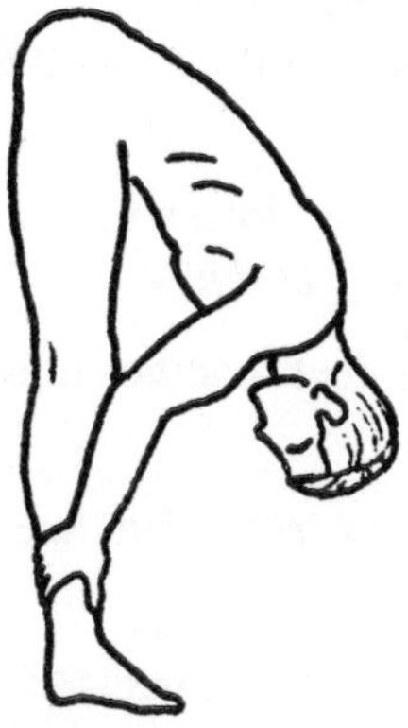

Figure 77. The Sun Worship Exercise.

3. Feel the warmth of the sunlight penetrate into the tissues.

NOTE: This exercise may be done lying down, but make sure that your sexual openings and anus are bathed in the sunlight.

LOWER BODY AND SEXUAL GLANDS EXERCISE

The primary symptoms of old age are often experienced as coldness or numbness in the legs and feet due to the deterioration of the circulatory system at the extremities of the body, stiffness of the joints, and lack of sexual energy. This exercise is designed to reverse these and other degenerative problems of the lower trunk, thus restoring youthfulness to the body. The pose increases the circulation to the toes, feet, and legs as well as the organs throughout the abdomen. It frees the pelvis and joints of the knees and ankles, strengthens the nerves throughout the lower trunk of the body, and stimulates the kidney, liver, and spleen-pancreas meridians which pass up on the inside of the legs and into the sexual glands. It works to cure sexual problems, such as impotence, premature ejaculation, and other problems of retardation. It also cures menstrual problems of the female system such as cramps and excessive bleeding. It is also an excellent exercise for pregnant women as it opens up the pelvis and assures an easy delivery.

1. Sit on the floor and bend your knees so that the soles of your feet come together in front of your body.

2. Rub the bottoms of your feet together until they are warm, and then touch them together.

3. Rub your toes with your fingers to stimulate the circulation in your feet.

4. With your feet together, draw your heels as close into the pelvis as you can set them.

5. Begin to work your knees down toward the floor by pressing your elbows in against your thighs while holding onto your toes with your hands. Do not force your knees down. Just allow the muscles to relax as you push them down.

6. Using the palms of your hands, rub the inside of your thighs starting at the knees, massaging upward to the inner pelvis. This will stimulate the liver, kidney, and spleen-pancreas meridians.

7. Repeat the massaging action for a total of 7 times.

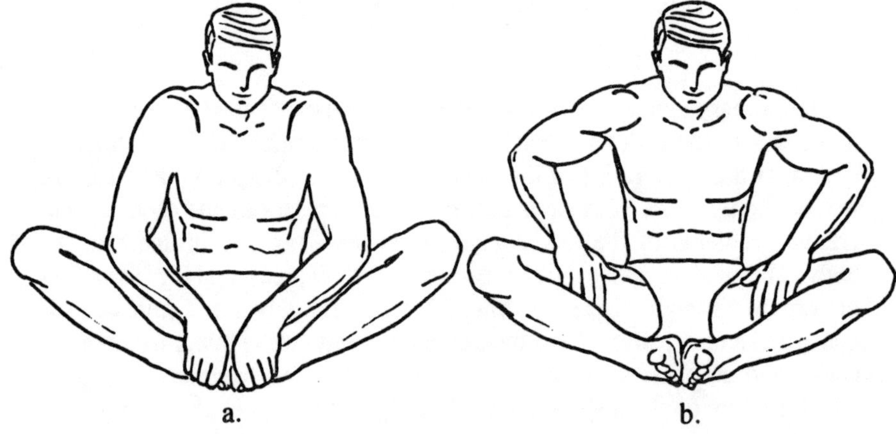

Figures 78a and 78b. Lower Body and Sexual Glands Exercise.

8. Then gently beat on your inner thighs with your fists. This will stimulate the circulation of blood and energy in your legs and sexual organs.

9. Continue to work with the exercise as long as you feel comfortable.

TOE WIGGLING AND BODY STRETCHING

During sleep, or for that matter during any prolonged period of inactivity, toxins accumulate in the muscles due to the decrease in circulation, which also results in stiffness. Old age is often said to begin in the toes, as older people often suffer from poor circulation and cold feet. What we need then is to stretch the body upon rising to help break up the toxins and restore the proper circulation to the muscles and tissues in the body. This helps us to wake up and become alert more quickly. If you observe animals such as the cat, you will see that when they wake up the first thing they do is stretch their bodies. They are following a natural law which we too need to follow.

1. Upon rising in the morning and while still in bed, stretch your arms, legs, back, and feet. It does not matter which way. Just stretch. Be very free about it, following no particular form or style. After you stretch, pause briefly to relax before getting up.

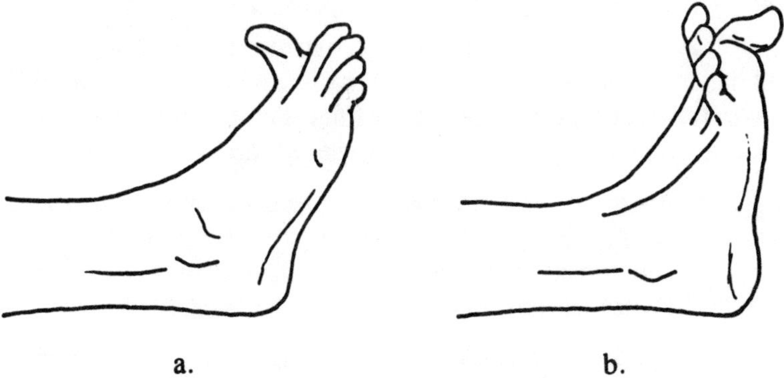

Figures 79a and 79b. Toe Wiggling Exercise.

2. Now you need to move and stimulate the toes. Wiggle the big toes back and forth several times. By moving the large toe, you stimulate all the nerves in the body.

3. Wiggle your toes twelve times. Make sure that you pay close attention to the toe movement, so that the exercise becomes a meditation as well. This will increase the benefits you derive from this exercise.

This is coincident to the science currently known as Reflexology. The related sciences of Reflexology and Zone Therapy have been known and practiced for over 6,000 years. When one wiggles the toes, the liver is exercised and stimulated and energy is sent to the sexual glands. By doing this exercise, you will have at one stroke stimulated your whole body through your feet.

INTERNAL ORGAN RELAXATION

The internal organs of four-legged animals hang freely within the abdomen, and so they are always assured the proper amount of blood. The organs of a human being, however, are piled one on top of the other when standing erect. We need, then, to give these organs a chance to relax and have some free space, so that they might enjoy proper circulation. Once again, we need to follow the example given to us by other animals. Begin this in the morning after stretching and wiggling the toes.

1. Roll over on your bed or onto the floor so that the toes, legs, knees, and hands are on the floor. You will be like a dog, with your head forward and your chest parallel to the floor. Pause a moment to allow blood to circulate freely into and around all the internal organs.

2. Then slowly sit back on your heels and lower your forehead toward the floor. Your arms will stretch out in front of you. Close your eyes and remain in this position for a few seconds, then come back to the kneeling position.

3. You may want to synchronize your breathing with the movements of the exercise, but however you do it, always keep the breathing easy and natural.

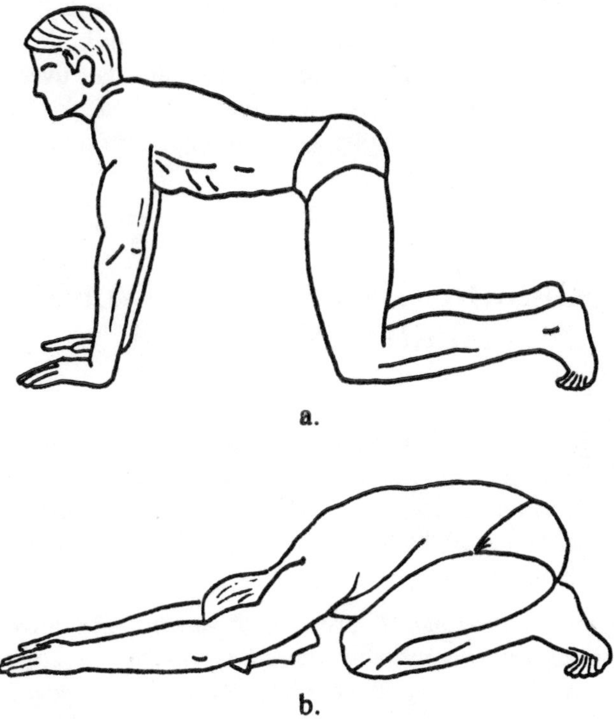

Figures 80a and 80b. Internal Organ Relaxation.

4. Repeat the exercise seven times.

In this exercise, blood is retained in the stomach and the intestines to strengthen digestion and elimination. Sitting down onto the heels forces blood to flow to the heart, lungs, and brain. Blood then flows back to the heart easily so that the heart has a chance to rest. During sound sleep, the flow of blood to the head is reduced. We need to start with this pose in the morning to bring the blood to our brain so that we will feel fresh, alert, and alive.

Those who have high blood pressure are cautioned not to practice this position until their blood pressure has been brought to within normal limits through the practice of the other Internal Exercises. This pose tends to bring too much blood to the brain and increases one's blood pressure, so that it may be dangerous for persons suffering from high blood pressure to perform this exercise.

It would also be wise for the average person to work into this pose gradually. One does not want to put such pressure on the brain too quickly. Allow the arteries, veins, and capillaries to accommodate over time to the increased flow of blood caused by this exercise. At first, practice the pose once or twice, slowly working up to seven times over a period of a few weeks.

RUBBING THE ARMS AND LEGS: MERIDIAN MASSAGE

Energy circulates throughout the body along minute pathways called *meridians*. An understanding of the meridians and their vital functions of providing every cell of the body with energy is mandatory if one is to master the techniques of the breathing and contemplation exercises in the system of Internal Exercises.

> *The means whereby man is created, the means whereby diseases occur, the means whereby man is cured, the means whereby diseases arise: the twelve meridians are the basis for all theory and treatment. The meridian is that which decides over life and death. Through it the hundred diseases may be treated.*
>
> Nei Ching

Regarding the meridians, Dr. Kim Bong Han of the University of Pyongang in North Korea, after conducting an extensive series of experiments, arrived at a conclusion for the actual existence of these pathways of energy. He reported that the meridians were actually composed of a type of histological tissue as yet unnoticed by scientists who, prior to Dr. Kim's experiments, had believed that the meridians were simply *imaginary* lines. He discovered the structure and function of the meridian system to be totally different from those of the lymphatic, circulatory, and nervous systems.

The meridians are symmetrical and bilateral channels with a diameter ranging between 20 and 50 millimicrons. They exist beneath the surface of the skin and have a thin membranous wall which is filled with a transparent, colorless fluid. Each of the main meridians develops intricate subsidiary branches, some of which supply adjacent areas with energy while others ultimately reach the surface of the skin. The places at which the branches reach the skin's surface are the points illustrated on an acupuncture chart. Often several branches from different main channels converge at a single point. By stimulating that point, the energy in several channels can be affected simultaneously. The meridians are encircled by blood vessels that are especially in abundance around the individual branches stemming from each of the main channels. (The bleeding that some patients report after undergoing acupuncture is an indication that the practitioner has narrowly missed the point on the surface of the skin and pierced one or many of the vascular vessels surrounding the point.)

After conducting many experiments, scientists discovered that the meridians are pathways for electricity. This led to the invention of a machine called the Point-Locator, an instrument which indicates the points where the branches of the meridians reach the skin's surface. At present, the quality of the impulse that travels along the meridians is the subject of intensive research among Chinese scientists, while many Western investigators are currently trying to determine possible associations between the meridians and the autonomic nervous system.

The meridian system, a physiological structure, provides a means by which many of the energy principles that have been labeled as purely hypothetical—even to the point where their actual existence has been questioned—can be proved valid. Since the reality of the meridian system has been experimentally verified by researchers like Dr. Kim, we can now conclude that the main functional purpose for which that system exists is to provide an effective means of transmitting the all-pervading but invisible energy which animates all manifestations of life. Their subtlety, when perceived in relationship to even the most microscopic aspects of the physical body, suggests that the meridians may well be the "missing link", or the threshold between pure energy and its first manifestations as microscopic matter.

Although the first scientific proof of the existence of the meridian system is believed to be the result of Dr. Kim's efforts, conclusive evidence for the existence of the meridians was found in 1937 by Sir Thomas Lewis of England. His report, published in the *British Medical Journal* of February, 1937, stated he had discovered an "unknown nervous system" that was unrelated to either the sensory or the sympathetic nervous systems. Rather than being composed of a network of nerves, he reported, the newly discovered system was composed of a network of incredibly minute lines.

Although his report went relatively unnoticed by his colleagues, it was the first concrete verification in the West of the physiological system that Taoists knew to exist thousands of years ago.

Meridian, a word borrowed from geography, indicates a line joining a series of ordered points. There are twelve main meridians. A meridian is assigned to each of the five organs, the six bowels, and the pericardium—here referred to as the Heart Constrictor. (The idea of the six bowels is often perplexing to those unacquainted with Taoist philosophy. The five organs are the heart, spleen-pancreas, lungs, kidneys, and liver. The six bowels are the large intestine, bladder, "Triple Heater" [an ancient term indicating the internal glandular system], gallbladder, small intestine, and stomach. The Heart Constrictor or pericardium corresponds to the blood vessel system. [Please refer to my book *The Great Tao* for a fuller explanation.])

Each of the main meridians has both a point of entry and a point of exit. Energy enters the meridian at the point of entry, circulates along the meridian, flows through the point of exit and on through the point of entry of the succeeding meridian. The point of exit on a meridian is connected to the point of entry on the succeeding meridian by a secondary channel. The direction of the flow of energy along a meridian remains constant and never vacillates after flowing through the point of entry. (See figures 83—96.)

The meridians are the means by which the organs and bowels are linked together, and by which each organ and bowel is enlivened by energy as it circulates along the meridian circuit. A question that might naturally arise as a result of the illustrations depicting the sequence of the main meridians is: "According to the information given thus far—if an organ or bowel associated with one of the main meridians were to become diseased, wouldn't it be logical to conclude that the energy would then be blocked and be unable to complete its cycle of circulation?" The answer is no, because in addition to the twelve main meridians, there are eight extraordinary meridians which provide for the circulation of energy when it becomes superfluous or excessive in one of the main meridians.

The eight extraordinary meridians can justifiably be called "lifesavers" in that they provide for bodily energy to continue its cycle of circulation, regardless of whether any one of the organs or bowels becomes diseased, thus blocking the meridian circuit. Taoist teachings explain the purpose of the eight extraordinary meridians as being analogous to the drainage ditches and dikes that sometimes exist alongside a major river (which, of course, corresponds to the major meridians). If for any reason the river should become flooded and overflow its banks, the drainage ditches are designed to accommodate the superfluous water. Just so, the flow of energy along the eight extraordinary meridians is not constant, but is determined by the amount of excess energy in the main meridian.

The meridians or energy channels which regulate the liver, pancreas, and kidneys all come together on the inside of the thighs. These three meridians come in to energize the entire upper channel of the body. By massaging these pathways correctly, we are able to stimulate the entire body, including the sexual organs, as these meridians pass through the pelvis on their way up the body. In a similar fashion, the gallbladder, bladder, and stomach meridians run in a downward path along the outside of the leg. By massaging these pathways, we stimulate the organs and tissues associated with the meridians.

Upward Massage

By massaging the legs on the inside in an upward manner, we stimulate the circulation of blood within the lower half of the body. People who have jobs which require them to sit or stand all day long tend to develop cramps and varicose veins in their legs. This is because the blood tends to gather in the feet and legs, which hampers proper circulation. By stimulating the meridians of the leg, we can strengthen the healthy flow of blood and prevent future problems from developing in the legs.

This exercise may be done standing, sitting, or lying down.

1. Place the palms of your hands on the inside of your legs at the ankles.

2. Slowly bring your palms up your legs, through the inside of your knees, up your thighs and into your genitals.

3. Repeat this movement for a total of 12 times.

NOTE: At all times keep pressure on your hands so that a slight warmth may be felt as you massage your leg. Breathe normally throughout the exercise. You may also practice this exercise by just concentrating on rubbing the area from the knee to the thigh. This is the most important part of the exercise.

Downward Massage

By massaging the outside of the legs in a downward fashion, problems such as high blood pressure, water retention, and obesity (all of which are associated with the gallbladder, bladder, and stomach meridians) can be corrected or prevented from occurring. Problems of bursitis and arthritis can also be reversed or at least prevented from degenerating further.

This exercise may be done standing, sitting, or lying down. The standing position also helps to stretch the hamstrings, knees, tendons, and calves of the legs and brings energy down into the toes.

1. Place the palms of your hands on the outside of your thighs.

2. In a continuous motion, rub your hands down your legs along the outside of your knees and calves until you come to the ankles.

3. Repeat this movement for a total of 12 times. Breathe normally as you perform the exercise.

This movement helps dispel the energy from the body. This is why it helps problems such as obesity, water retention, and high blood pressure. You will want to do this in the morning as at that time it is preferable to energize the body by practicing the upward massage only.

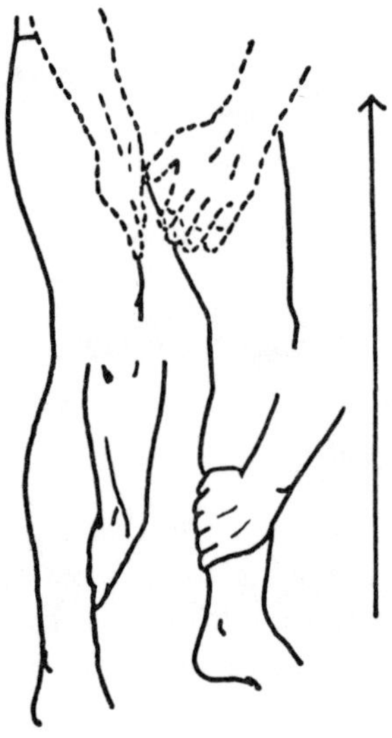

a. Upward Meridians.

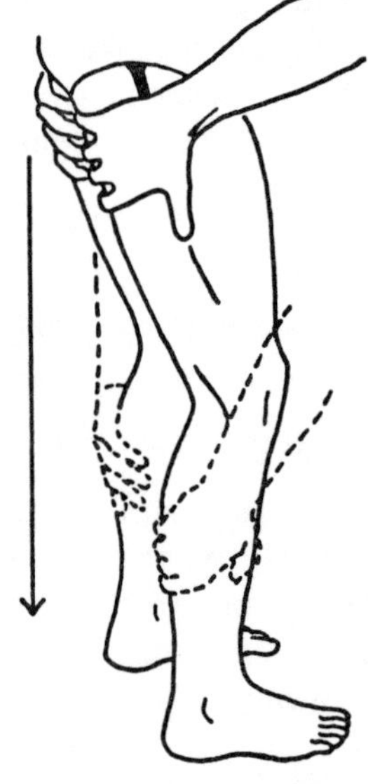

b. Downward Meridians.

Figures 81a and 81b. Meridian Massage: Leg Rubbing.

Arm Massage

Just as with the leg massage, you may massage your arms to stimulate the heart, lung, and Heart Constrictor meridians which run down the inside of the arm and the Triple Heater, large intestine, and small intestine meridians which run up on the outside of the arms toward the shoulders.

1. Place your left palm on the inside of your right shoulder.

2. In a continuous motion, rub your palm down through the inside of your elbow to the tips of your fingers.

3. Bring your left palm over your fingers and continue to rub up the back of your hand, through the outside of your elbow and onto your shoulder.

4. Repeat this movement for a total of 12 times.

5. Reverse the above by bringing your right hand onto your left arm, rubbing first downward on the inside of the arms, then upward along the outside of the arms. Repeat this also for a total of 12 times.

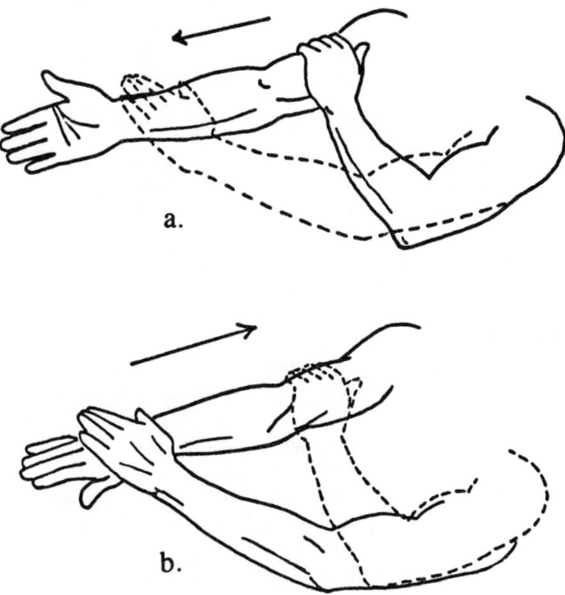

Figures 82a and 82b. Meridian Massage: Arm Rubbing.

The efficacy of the Internal Exercises is based on the development of the proper flow of energy throughout the meridians in the body. Each exercise is designed to stimulate a particular meridian, or, as in the case of the Meridian Meditation, the entire meridian system. By learning the Internal Exercises, especially the Meridian Massage, we are able to help our bodies gain control over the very energy upon which all life depends. We can then use this energy to heal both ourselves and others, and to insure our continuing health and spiritual growth and even our potential immortality.

PART III

ADVANCED LIVING

7

Taoist Meditative, Contemplative, and Breathing Exercises

In addition to the physical exercises, the ancient Taoists discovered invaluable methods of meditation and breathing, such as the Meridian Meditation, Brain Cleansing and Breathing Exercises. They used these to augment the energy within their bodies, to help provide for a constant and unimpeded flow of energy along the meridians, as well as providing a tool for observing inner states of weakness and disease. They also discovered practical contemplative exercises, such as the North Star Meditation, Candlelight and Sunlight Contemplations, and Concentration Exercise, which were used to focus their energy in desired directions toward specific goals, such as a new job or financial security or to cultivate the mind or peace of mind.

The Taoists developed meditative breathing techniques which were concerned with transmuting the flow of the generative energy. Instead of being discharged to procreate offspring or to waste away, it is retained in the body for purification and transmutation into positive vitality. These techniques, called Immortal Breathing (the Small and Large Heavenly Cycles), are a series of comprehensive methods designed to create an alchemical change within the practitioner to bring him or her into a final state of self-realization and immortality.

The Taoist exercises, including the physical, meditative, contemplative, and breathing techniques, are aimed at the unification of the spirit, mind, and body. If an individual is forever unified in mind, body, and spirit, he or she will never die, for death is a separation of spirit and body. Unification is the way of God, or life, and separation is the way of Satan, or death. With these principles in mind, one can isolate true teachings from the false: those which are true will promote life, and those which are false will promote separation of spirit and body. Upon practicing the Internal Exercises the practitioner will immediately recognize the exercises as being the former, for friction between the spirit, mind, and body will be reduced until there is only complete unification, oneness, and stillness—the realization of Tao.

The first step in all the Internal Exercises encourages the practitioner to do something, to take some kind of action either through specific physical or concentrative tasks. Then these will enable the practitioner to go beyond action into the Tao, or a state of action without action. The practice of the breathing and meditative aspects of the Internal Exercises leads one into a realization of this second step—that of non-action.

According to Taoist theory, realizing the Tao occurs in three stages. The first stage is called *you wei*, meaning "action", or diligent practice. By working hard, we will arrive at the higher stage, which in Chinese is called *wu wei*, meaning "no action". At this point we need not attend to everything personally in order to do everything. However, for the entering into the Tao to occur, we must learn that in every state of non-action there is action, in order to enter into the highest stage, called *wu bu wei*, where everything is done without any need for action.

In the pursuit of learning, every day something is acquired.
In the pursuit of the Tao, every day something is dropped.
Less and less is done
Until non-action is achieved.
When nothing is done, nothing is left undone.
The world is ruled by letting things take their course.
It cannot be ruled by interfering.

Tao Te Ching XLVIII

By practicing the Internal Exercises, man prepares himself for this final transformation which occurs in a state beyond time and space, in which man realizes his true natural place in the universe.

MERIDIAN MEDITATION

Utilizing the pathways of energy which already exist in the body, Meridian Meditation enables its practitioner to turn her/his eyes inward to her/his own body and detect states of weakness as if she/he were seeing them clearly with her/his eyes. Once properly versed in this discipline, no one will be better equipped than you to diagnose your own state of physical health.

Modern day machines and analytical techniques (X-rays, scanners, blood and urine analysis, etc.) are useful in diagnosing certain diseases, especially inflammatory diseases, but they have more problems diagnosing degenerative diseases related to nerve and energy problems which subtly weaken organs and tissues and later lead to complex medical problems. These problems are detected only when it is too late. Weakness *is* the first step toward disease. If we have no weaknesses, then it will be impossible to contract a serious illness. Through the technique of Meridian Meditation we are able to enter into our own energy pathways and detect any illness before it is too late. Then when we discover a problem such as an energy blockage, we can use the different modes of healing available to us, such as Internal Exercises, herbs, Tui-Na, etc.

Meridian Meditation can often be used to uncover the origins of a weakness first thought to be located in another point in the body. A case in point is illustrated by the time I was plagued with a harsh and constant cough which was irritating the mucous linings in my throat, thus making it exceedingly difficult for me to talk. At first I thought this was due to a problem within the lungs and took appropriate herbs to treat what I thought to be the source of my problem. When the irritation still did not disperse, I suspected something else might be wrong. Using the Meridian Meditation, I observed that the origin of the problem was not in my lungs, but in my heart, the organ which supports the lungs. And so, after using a different set of herbs to treat the heart, the cough began to abate the next day. The Meridian Meditation can also be practiced as a preventive technique. It gives the student a method to discern states of weakness before they become major diseases. For example, cancer takes many years to manifest into its outward form. The inner observation one gains through Meridian Meditation can help prevent it at its onset. Thus, this method of self-diagnosis helps a person to see all the signs before a disease begins to take hold in the body.

Meridian Meditation is also a system of self-healing. By meditating on sites within the body where energy has become blocked, it is possible to re-establish an unimpeded flow of energy at this point. For thousands of years, Meridian Meditation has been used for this purpose, and it has contributed greatly to the physical and spiritual development of many Taoist sages.

Meridian Meditation is learned in three stages: 1. Memorizing the meridians, 2. Feeling the energy pathways, and 3. Tracing all twelve meridians at once.

1. First you must familiarize yourself with the meridians. To do this thoroughly and accurately, you should buy a good acupuncture chart. Learn them one at a time, in the prescribed sequence as they are illustrated in the figures. The first meridian will be the lung meridian. To reinforce its memory, use the bulb of the thumb or the tips of the index and middle fingers to gently massage the entire length of the meridian. As you do this follow the correct direction of the flow of energy. Go up where the energy flows up and go down where it flows down.

2. After becoming thoroughly acquainted with the paths of the meridian and the direction of energy flow, try to feel the energy flow within the meridians. The correct method is to first find a comfortable position, either lying or sitting down. Sitting on a soft cushion is preferable; keep the spinal column straight so that the tail bone and the spinal column at the waist are in line. Your shoulders and back should be relaxed, however, so that the shoulders automatically fall into their natural position, which is slightly forward. This allows for maximum expansion of the lungs. Place the hands on the legs with the thumbs folded inside the palms. Empty the mind of all irrelevant, excess thoughts and focus all of your attention upon the lung meridian. You may want to begin by tracing the path of the lung meridian with your fingers, as in stage 1. Now pay close attention to the subjective feeling that arises as a result of this procedure. Then keep your hands

on your legs and try to feel a flow of energy descend down your arm along the lung meridian. Eventually you will sense even the most minute energy fluctuations along the meridian. Continue to repeat this procedure along the large intestine meridian and subsequent meridians in their appropriate order. After a number of practice sessions, you will begin to perceive the flow of energy along the meridians.

3. When you are able to feel the flow of energy in all twelve meridians, you will want to do many meridians at the same time. For instance, you may want to do all the meridians that pass through the head, the torso, or the lower half of the body at once. To do so many at once, you should first assume the body position described for stage 2. Cleanse the mind of all irrelevant, excess thoughts and focus all of your attention upon the meridians in the head. You may begin tracing the meridians by holding your entire hand over the meridians. Do this slowly and pay close attention to the subjective feelings that arise. Feel for energy flows. Continue to repeat this procedure until you sense even the most minute energy fluctuations in the head. Repeat this procedure for all the meridians in the torso and the lower half of the body.

NOTE A: Occasionally, as you begin your practice, you will sense an energy blockage where it will be difficult to follow the energy along the particular meridian you are tracing. For example, you may feel the energy flowing down the arm on the lung meridian, but it may stop when you get to the elbow. Thus you will know that you have a blockage of some sort. Begin again at the upper arm and retrace the flow. If it blocks again, begin again until you feel an unimpeded flow of energy. This may take several attempts or it may take weeks to get past this area. However, when you do feel that the energy is flowing smoothly and freely, you will know that you have effectively prevented or corrected a weakness or disease within yourself. If the energy does not flow properly after a number of attempts at one sitting, go on to feel out the flow of energy throughout the other meridians. Then, either when you have finished or at another sitting, you may return to the energy block.

NOTE B: Always keep in mind what you are doing. If the mind wanders, then start again from the beginning. Do not be anxious to hurry the process. First feel where the energy is going and do not interrupt your feeling process. Eventually you will be able to very directly feel the flow of energy.

With the Meridian Meditation, in as little as three months, one will be able to willfully feel the energy flow along any one of the meridians. Becoming consciously aware of the circulation of energy within the body will enable one to maintain a state of energy balance under any and all circumstances. Disease can only inhabit a body in which there is an erratic flow of energy along the meridians.

We need to learn to make our way around the inner world before we can learn to make our way around the universe. By practicing this method of meditation, one will learn how to unify the mind and the body in one's personal microcosm. Then it will be possible to "know" the universal macrocosm that lies beyond our apparent limitations, the goal that is attained when we have reached the Tao.

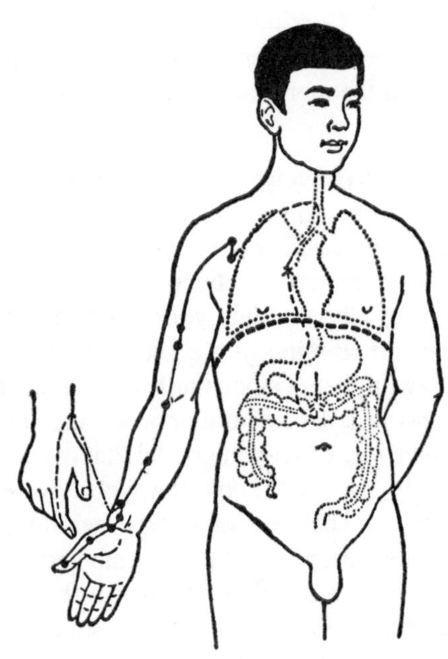

Figure 83. Lung Meridian.

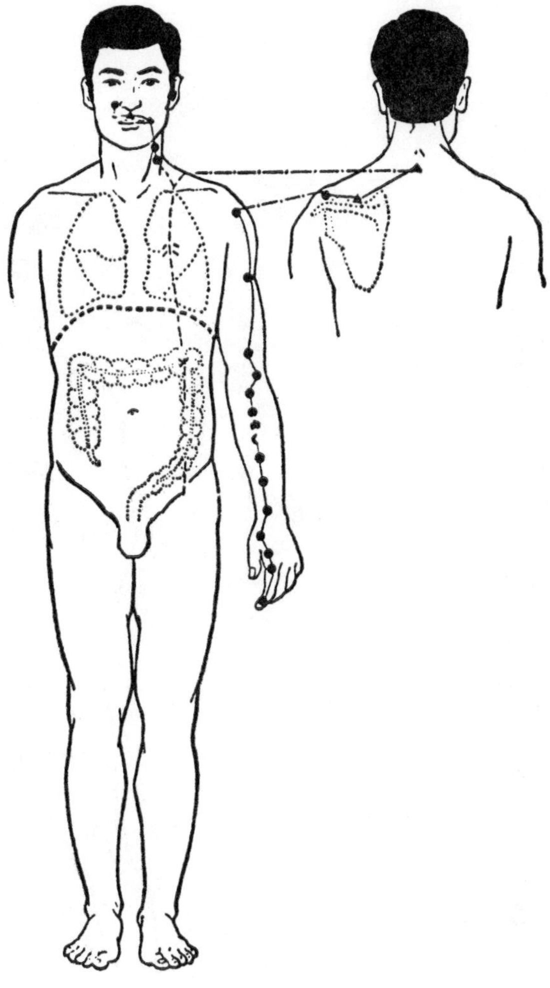

Figure 84. Large Intestine Meridian

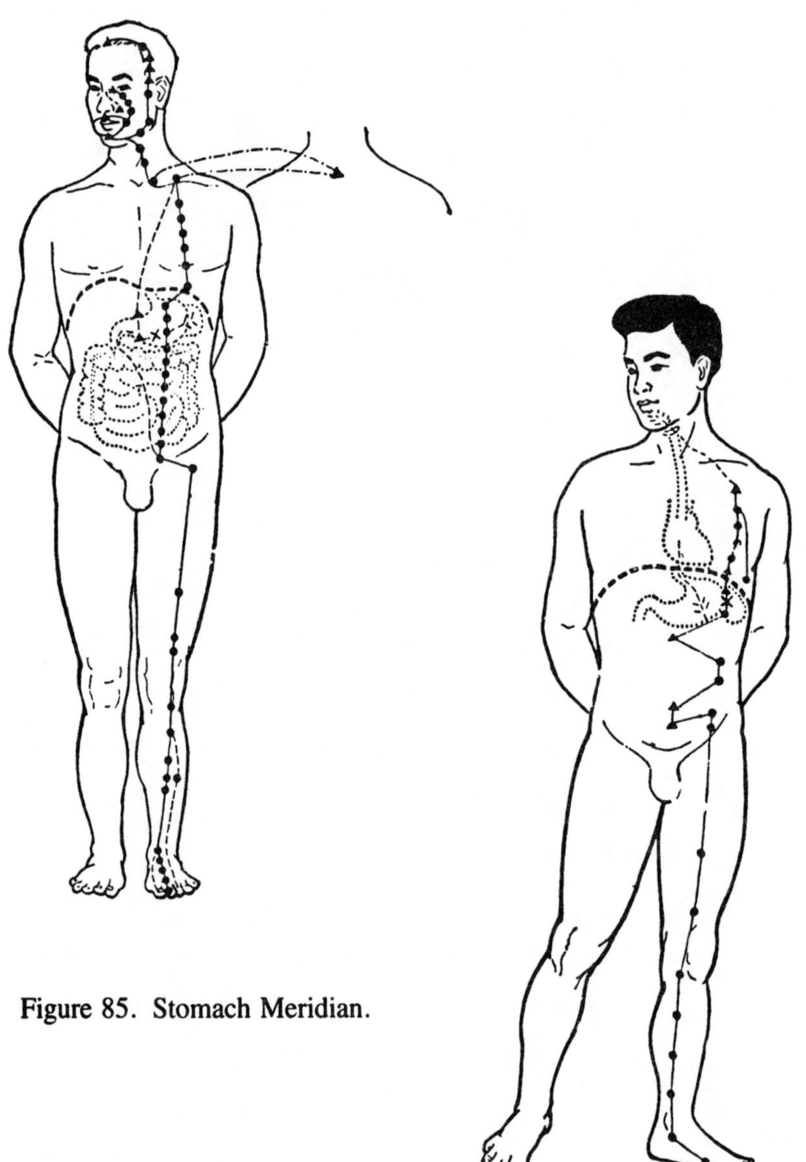

Figure 85. Stomach Meridian.

Figure 86. Spleen-Pancreas Meridian.

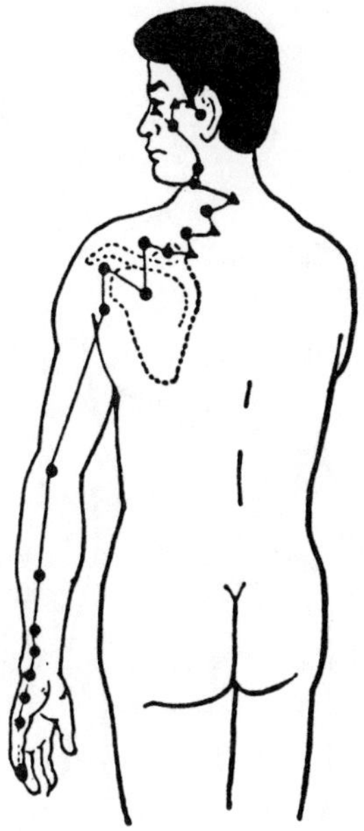

Figure 88.
Small Intestine Meridian.

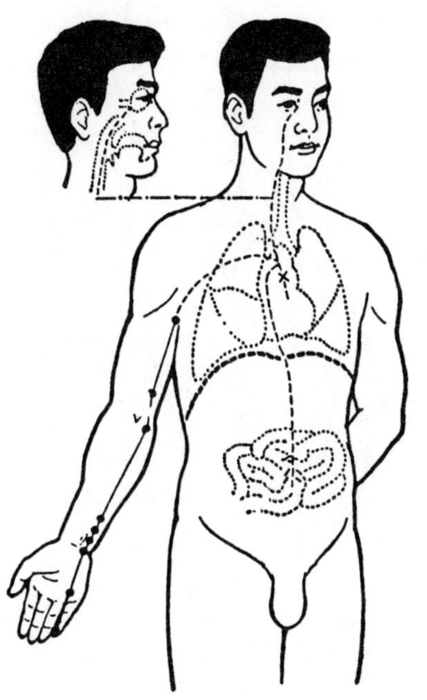

Figure 87. Heart Meridian.

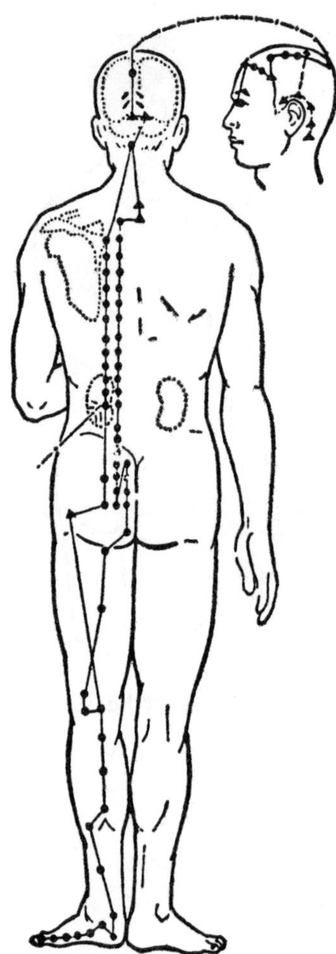

Figure 89. Bladder Meridian.

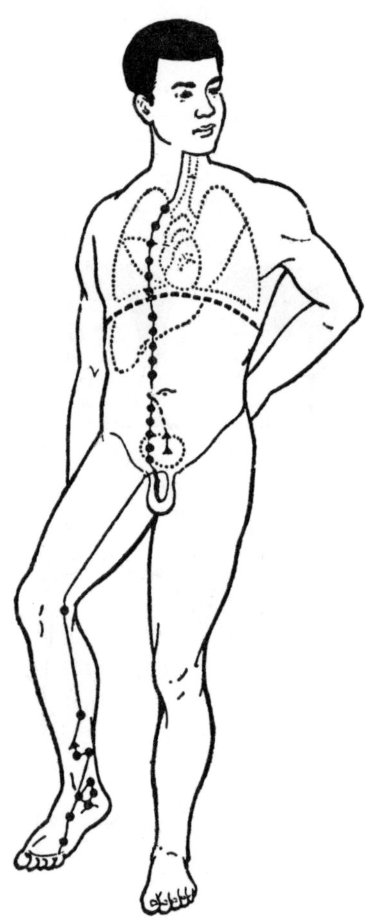

Figure 90. Kidney Meridian.

Figure 92.

Triple Heater Meridian.

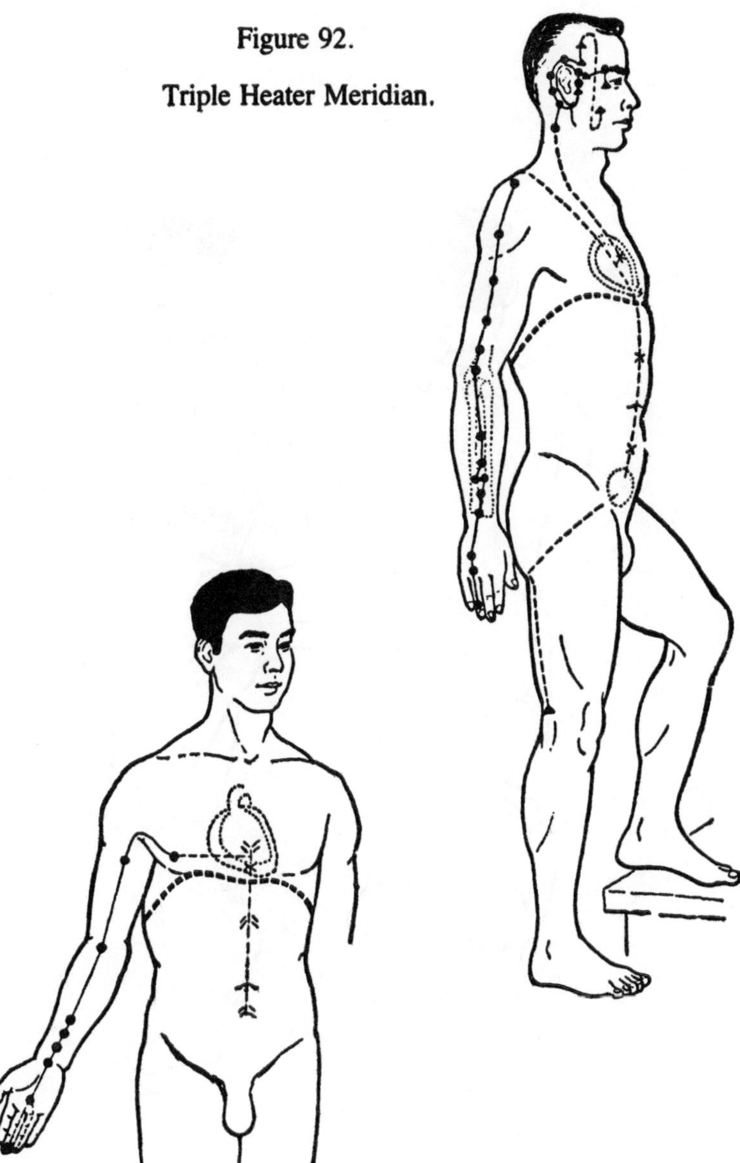

Figure 91. Heart Constrictor Meridian.

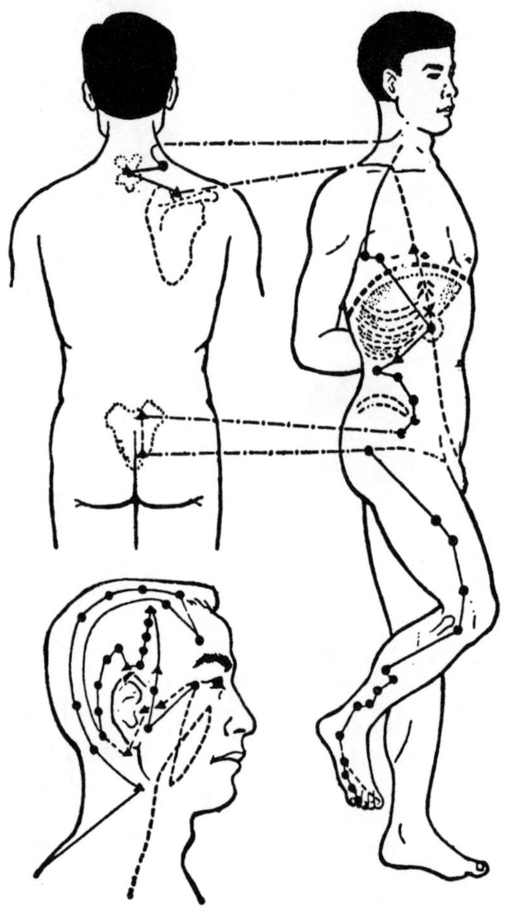

Figure 93. Gallbladder Meridian.

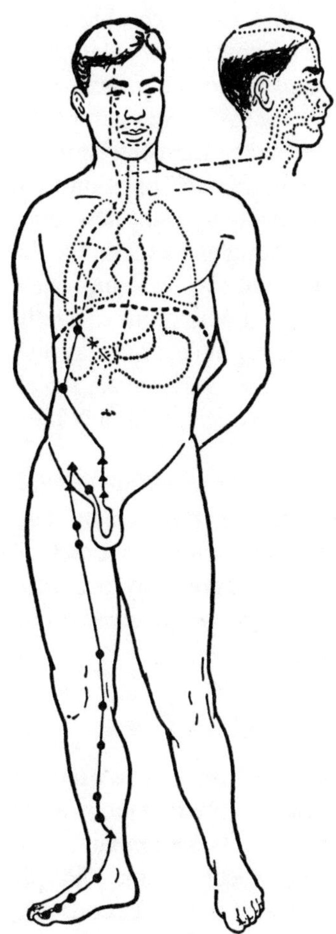

Figure 94. Liver Meridian.

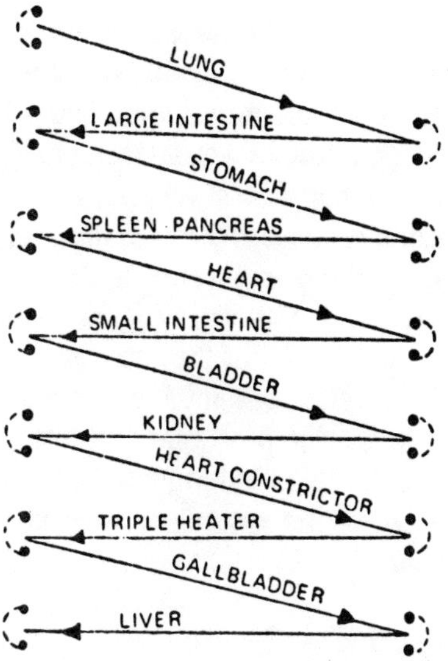

LUNG
LARGE INTESTINE
STOMACH
SPLEEN PANCREAS
HEART
SMALL INTESTINE
BLADDER
KIDNEY
HEART CONSTRICTOR
TRIPLE HEATER
GALLBLADDER
LIVER

Figure 95.

Sequence of Energy Flow.

MEDITATIVE AND CONTEMPLATIVE EXERCISES

A person may practice the North Star Meditation, Candlelight, Sunlight, or Moonlight Contemplations, and Concentration Exercise for practical as well as healing purposes. These contemplative exercises help those who are in need of a job, health, money, intelligence, or love. For example, if one wants to find a new job, one would imagine that the light entering into one's head *is* the new job. One would put all wishes and hopes into the meditation. It is not necessary to even know specifically what the new job is to be. If one is able to correctly perform the meditation and experience the golden light throughout one's body, a new job will be awaiting one's acceptance. In a similar manner, one may fill oneself with money, intelligence, happiness, love, or any other need that one may have. One may also achieve success through the practice of the Concentration Exercise, which strengthens and trains one's mind to overcome weaknesses that may keep success at bay.

As with all of the Internal Exercises, and the breathing and meditation techniques, one must experience them to understand and appreciate their simple, yet profound, effects. The ancient Taoists were very practical people. If something worked well, they used it. If it did not, they discarded it. And this system of Internal Exercise has been in use for over 6,000 years!

North Star Meditation

The North Star is the guide star of the heavens and has been used for centuries by travelers to pinpoint their location and ensure that their routes of travel were correct. It has been called "The King", "The Emperor", or the "Highest Place", and it has been given the special name "Purple Rose" because of its beautiful purple aura. Further, it is forever constant, forever hovering over the earth and therefore forever dependable. So it is fitting that the Taoists have used it for thousands of years in a meditative exercise they use for healing and other beneficial purposes.

The best time to practice this meditation is in the evening when you are able to see the North Star clearly. However, it may be performed during the daytime by simply imagining that the star is there above you. However, always face the North Star when you are practicing this exercise. It will then be easy for your body to accept and receive the electromagnetic energy coming from the star.

1. Begin by sitting facing the North Star, which may be located by first finding the Big Dipper.

2. Use your imagination and feel the light of the North Star come down and meet you on the top of your head at a place called "The Meeting of All Points". This point lies at the crown of the head at a point equidistant between the ears.

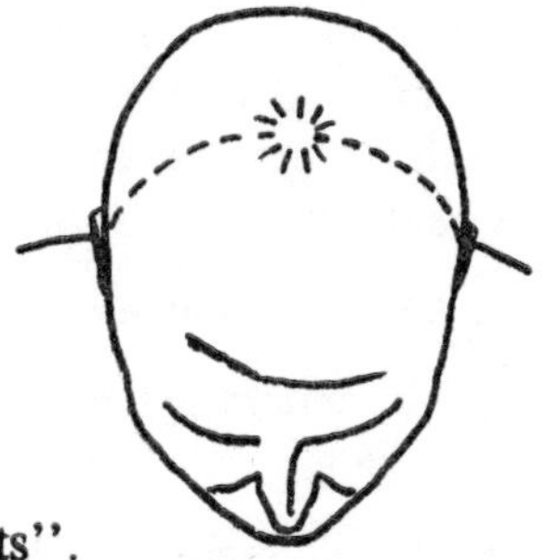

Figure 96.
The "Meeting of All Points".

3. Feel the energy from the "Purple Rose" meet your energy at this point, and imagine that this area of your head produces a golden fire. The meridians of your body will begin to look transparent and golden. Feel the golden light penetrate throughout your entire body and down to the toes.

NOTE: If is often extremely difficult to practice this exercise, as you need complete attention on what you are doing for it to be successful. If your attention wanders or you are interrupted, start again. However, never force yourself to perform the meditation. If you are unable to complete it successfully, stop and come back to it another time. Eventually you will meet with success. Once you are able to complete the meditation and feel the golden light enter your body, you may discover that some places within your body will appear dark, while all the rest remains a golden color. The dark area within your body is a disease. Allow the light from the North Star to soak into this dark area until this place also becomes transparent and golden. Then you will be charged with energy and your diseases will be healed.

Whenever you have a disease, you may use this exercise to literally wash it away. It works. "As you think, so you will be." You will also find that it helps to refresh, heal, and strengthen your body.

Candlelight, Sunlight, and Moonlight Contemplations

If you are unable to locate the North Star, you may practice the exercise using a candle. You may also use the sun or the moon as the source of the golden light which you wish to absorb into your body. But you should take into consideration the facts that the sun may be too hot and the moon may be too cold. You can start using the Candlelight, Sunlight, and Moonlight Contemplations to heal yourself today, whereas the Meridian Meditation may take several months to learn.

The contemplations may be done in the early mornings, just before sunset, or on a cold day.

1. Look at a candle or the source of light.

2. Close you eyes and bring the light into your head. Feel your head fill with golden light.

3. Then, feel the light gradually fill your neck, shoulders, trunk, and entire body.

NOTE A: When performing the Candlelight or Moonlight Contemplations, face north and sit in a comfortable position. Do not face north when you do the Sunlight Contemplation and do not sit in the sun for longer than 10 minutes, as sunlight is strong and the earth's magnetic force flows from north to south.

NOTE B: The candle is the best source of light. It is best not to substitute a candle with an electric light bulb.

NOTE C: If some blockage comes in when you do the contemplation, open your eyes, gaze at the candle, and start over again. Do so until you can fill your entire body with transparent light. If someone sees you, he or she will think light is projecting out from your body. When you get proficient at filling your body with light, you may see some dark places which are not filled by light. These are diseased areas which can be healed if you work on them by filling them with light.

Concentration Exercise

To make one's way through life successfully, one must train one's mind to make proper use of its powers. How often have you heard or read that concentration is the main reason why some people are able to do everything well? The ancient Taoists were very aware of the connection between concentration and betterment, so they created the Concentration Exercise to strengthen the powers of concentration.

The exercise is done by concentrating on one of three points of focus: the point called *Ying Tang* (located on the forehead between the eyebrows, or at the level of the third eye), the point called *Shan Chung* (located at the thymus gland), and the point called *Chi Hai* (located 1 1/2 inches below the navel). You may use the figure below to find the points, or you may locate the points on an acupuncture chart. (If you choose the latter alternative, look for points #17 and #6 on the *Jen-Mo* meridian. However, you will not find the equivalent of point *Ying Tang* on the chart because that point is an extra point on the *Jen-Mo* meridian.) Sometimes the three points are called, from top to bottom, the upper *Tan Tien*, middle *Tan Tien*, and lower *Tan Tien*.

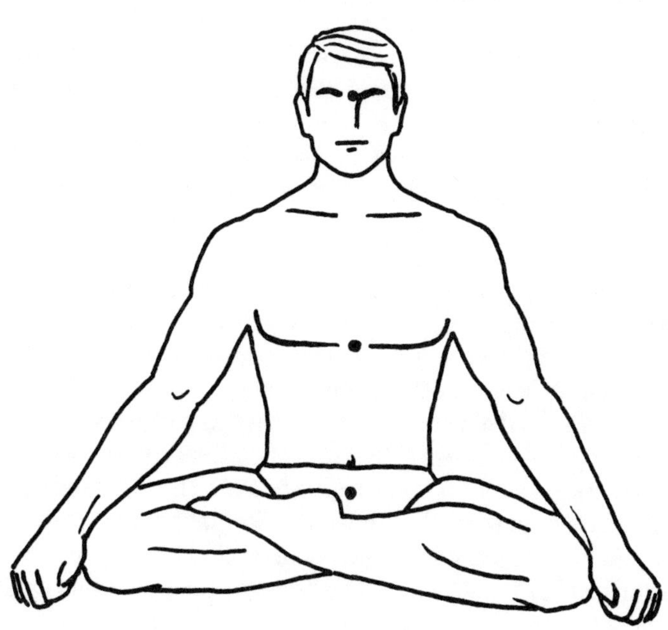

Figure 97. The *Ying Tang*, *Shan Chung*, and *Chi Hai* points.

This exercise may be done in the prone, sitting, or standing position whenever you have a quiet period of time to yourself.

1. You may begin by sitting with your legs crossed on a flat surface.

2. Now concentrate on one of the three points illustrated in figure 97. The point most often selected for this purpose is point *Chi Hai*. Concentrate by thinking only of this point and by removing any extra thoughts. Concentrate until heat is felt at that point.

3. Once you are able to feel the heat, discontinue and forget the exercise. You have succeeded in accomplishing this difficult exercise, and you may apply your concentrative abilities to other areas of your life.

NOTE: Do not be discouraged if the first few trials yield no results. This is a difficult exercise, and it may take several weeks before heat can be felt by some people. But once you feel the heat, you should forget about the exercise. Continuing to do the exercise to experience the sensations can cause serious damages.

The difficulty of this exercise is shown by the many mental aids people use to help themselves concentrate. Some recommend combining the exercise with breathing exercises— then air may be visualized to travel to the point of focus to heat the area. Others recommend manipulating the point or visualizing fires burning at the point. But once they have surpassed the difficulty and experienced the heat, their hearts will be filled with elation.

Unfortunately, this feeling of elation buries some people, especially the superstitious and uneducated, in self-conceit and encourages them to abuse the exercise. What is just a simple metabolic reaction in the body (concentrating on a point brings more circulation to the point of focus, and heightened activity in that area causes the sensations of warmth) is thought to be a working of the gods or a generation of godlike powers. Being able to achieve such a sensation boosted these people's egos tremendously.

Unfortunately, opportunistic cult leaders saw in this way of thinking an opportunity to control the simple-minded masses, so they created a variation of the original exercise. This variation encourages constant concentration to generate heat (energy) in the navel area and constant concentration to send that energy directly to any corner of the body. By teaching this exercise to unsuspecting people, cult leaders were able to generate a large following. Their followers were told that constant and ritualized use of this exercise, and only this exercise, gave them godly powers that could immediately make them impervious to all lethal weapons and all diseases and make them great and immortal at the same time. So whenever the followers needed a psychological lift, they would generate some heat in the abdomen and then use their *minds* to send the heat (energy) directly from the abdomen to the sexual organs or any other place in the body at will, in order to become "holy", to feel elated or energitic, or become "immortal" (even though they had no idea what the characteristics of energy were). As a result many died from the lack of proper medical care, mental and physical illnesses (caused by misguided interference with the delicate workings of the body), robbing raids led by cult leaders (the followers were beholden to their leaders for making them immortal, so they willingly did what their leaders demanded), rebellions (also led by cult leaders), and executions (in the hands of the local magistrates).

By researching the historical records, one can trace the development of a simple exercise into a cause of widespread chaos and mental illness among the poor and illiterate. These records show that the altered form of the exercise causes loss of appetite, hallucinations, uncontrolled shaking and trembling of the entire body (nerve damage), impotence, infertility, accelerated aging, cancers, schizophrenia, and moral corruption (incests, promiscuity, murders, and so on). The cult members were like walking time-bombs, and because their conditions were incurable, the local magistrates were required by law to execute them.

The powerful mind, like a nuclear bomb, must be handled carefully. Over-concentration can lead to imbalance. Since Taoism stresses that balance is the key to mental and physical health, anything that is overused is capable of causing imbalance and is therefore distinct from true Taoism. True Taoists teach that the Concentration Exercise is learned in two steps:

1. CONCENTRATING
2. FORGETTING

You are probably already familiar with such a process. For instance, when you first learned how to ride a bicycle, you had to concentrate very hard to balance yourself, otherwise an accident would occur. Then, when your riding skills improved so much that you rode as if you were walking, you naturally forgot to concentrate; otherwise, mulling over every movement at that advanced stage would cause a big accident.

BREATHING EXERCISES

There are many kinds of breathing besides the regular, in/out breathing of normal, everyday life. One of these—the Crane breathing—has been explained earlier. Other techniques include the following exercises. All of these exercises bring about a myriad of health benefits, including the ability to last 50% longer during demanding physical performances such as ballet, gymnastics, etc.

The Reverse Crane I

This exercise allows thorough gaseous exchange to take place in the lung and stomach tissues because it passes the air slowly throughout the lungs and stomach. Such thorough exchanges of oxygen and carbon dioxide usually do not occur with the regular method of breathing.

This exercise may be practiced in the mornings or evenings while standing, sitting, or while assuming a prone position.

1. Begin by exhaling slowly. As you do this, pull the stomach in so that air is pushed out of the stomach and the lungs. You want to imagine that every drop of air is leaving the stomach and lungs.

2. After you exhale completely, begin to inhale slowly and extend the lungs outward so that your chest expands in all directions. Try not to allow the stomach to expand—pull it in tightly. You want to use only the muscles in the chest while doing the first half of this exercise.

3. When the lungs are full, hold your breath for a while, to prevent the air from escaping from or entering into the lungs, and to allow full gaseous exchange to take place.

4. Next, slowly pull your chest in to contract the lungs. As you do so, slowly push out your stomach so that it becomes like a balloon. This series of actions pushes the air out of the lungs and into the stomach.

5. After retaining the air in the abdomen for a while, slowly contract the stomach and let the air out directly from the mouth. At first the exercise may be difficult to do, but with continued practice, you will be able to fill and empty the abdomen quite easily.

6. One complete inhale followed by an exhale comprises one round of breathing. At first, you will only be able to perform two or three

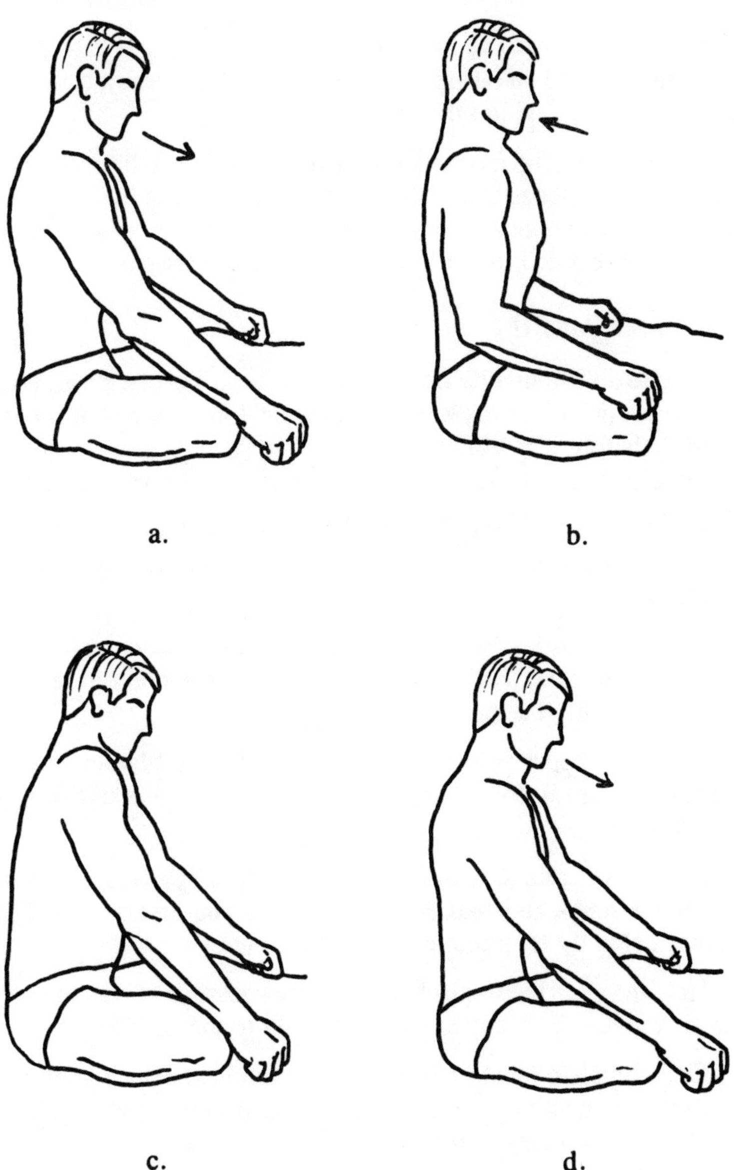

Figures 98a — 98d. Reverse Crane I.

rounds of breathing at one sitting. Eventually you want to perform twelve rounds. Always remember to do the exercise slowly.

NOTE: Women are cautioned not to perform this exercise during pregnancy as the in/out motions of the abdomen may create unpleasant feelings within the abdomen.

Besides allowing full oxygenation and invigoration of the bodily tissues, this exercise also tones abdominal tissues and enlarges the chest. It also encourages deeper regular breathing and full elimination of stagnant gases that are often retained in the lower portion of the lungs.

The Reverse Crane II

This exercise differs slightly from the first in these repects: the air is drawn into the upper portion of the lungs and later held in the stomach for as long as possible before it is exhaled.

This exercise may be done in any position, at any time of day.

1. Begin exhaling slowly by pulling in the stomach muscles. Use the stomach and diaphragm to squeeze every bit of air out of the stomach and lungs.

2. After you exhale completely, begin to inhale slowly to expand and fill the entire upper portion of the lungs. Keep the stomach in—you want to use only the muscles of the upper lungs.

3. When the upper portion of the lungs is full, hold your breath a while to prevent air from escaping and to allow full gaseous exchange to take place.

4. Now slowly pull the chest in to contract the lungs. Squeeze the air out of the lungs and into the stomach. As you do so expand the stomach slightly to accommodate the inflow of air.

5. Hold the air in the stomach for as long as possible. Then slowly let the air out the stomach. Exhale it directly to the outside.

6. One complete inhale followed by a complete exhale comprises one round of breathing. You may do as many rounds as you wish, but you should not carry it to an excess.

NOTE: At first you may not be able to hold the air inside the stomach very long. But with practice, you will be able to hold the air for a long time. Also, when you do the exercise, try to decelerate the inhalations and exhalations so that the stream of air will not even stir the hairs of the nostrils. These techniques will make you appear calm and strong through any rigorous activity, since you will not need to hyperventilate for air.

Using this technique during strenuous external exercise will improve your performance by as much as fifty percent. It supplies the body with all the oxygen and energy it needs throughout any rigorous performance as it eliminates the signs of hyperventilation, beautifying any performance tremendously. So the person who uses this technique will not tire easily, even after hours of non-stop activity. For these reasons, the breathing technique was adopted by the Oslo Ballet School in Norway. Gymnasts who have adopted this technique experienced a tremendous improvement in their performance. Research done on the effects of the technique upon athletes during their routines showed that their lasting power increased by as much as 50%.

Bone Breathing

We need a certain amount of tension to live, as the total absence of tension means death. However, it is a medical fact that excessive tension and stress cause disease, quite probably even cancer. Taoists have understood for centuries that the best way to protect against disease is to give oneself a full body and mind relaxation at least once a day. Relaxation is of the utmost importance for proper healing to take place, as it helps prevent energy blocks caused by the build-up of tension.

1. Lie on your back with your feet slightly apart, your arms next to your body, and your palms turned slightly upward. Allow the floor or bed to support the weight of your body rather than using your muscles to hold you up. Keep your eyes closed and let your breathing become regular.

2. As you inhale, feel the fresh, clean air and energy and vitality enter into and penetrate your entire body.

3. As you exhale, feel all the toxins and stale air leave your body.

4. Now begin to feel, as you inhale, the air as it comes in through your toes, flows up through the bones of your leg, and enters into your chest.

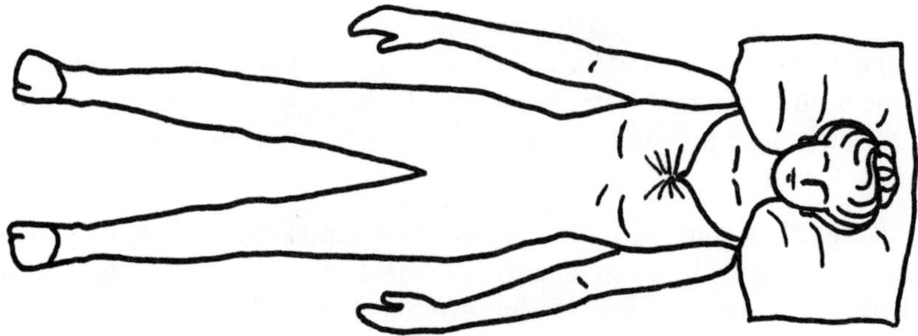

Figure 99. Bone Breathing.

5. As you breathe out, imagine feeling the air descend through the chest, pass through your leg and out through the toes of your foot.

6. Repeat steps 5 and 6 for a total of three times with each leg.

7. Now imagine feeling the air come up through your hands and arms and enter into your chest and head.

8. On the exhale, follow the air back down through your arm and out through your hand.

9. Repeat steps 7 and 8 for a total of three times with each arm.

NOTE A: Once you have mastered the individual movements, you may combine the flow of the breath through both arms and legs simultaneously.
NOTE B: If it is not practical to assume a prone position (at work or traveling, for example), then close your eyes and practice the exercise in a sitting position with your spine as straight as possible, and your arms and legs in a relaxed and comfortable position.

After completing the Bone Breathing exercise, your mind and body will feel completely rested and relaxed, and you will feel refreshed and ready to begin your work anew.

Energizing and Relaxing Breathing Exercises

Bodily energy is divided into Yin energy and Yang energy. Yin energy is negative, calm, and sedative in nature. Yang energy is positive, stimulative, and tonic.

These energies are related to sympathetic and parasympathetic nervous impulses and ion generation. When the sympathetic nervous system is activated, Yang energy increases. With its increase, blood pressure, heartbeat, breathing, sexual desire, etc. increase. Meanwhile, the body also generates positive ions. Because of the rise in positive ion levels, people experience headaches, hypertension, stress, tension, and so on. In contrast, when Yin energy increases, negative ions are generated. Together these stimulate the parasympathetic nervous system, resulting in decreased blood pressure, slower heartbeat and breathing, decreased sexual desire, and so on. Excessive Yin energy results in drowsiness, depression, sadness, weakness, etc.

Hence, the human body is an ion generator that generates both positive and negative ions. But it must generate these ions in a balanced manner, otherwise daily living will be uncomfortable.

How does one adjust or balance Yin and Yang energies?

Simply by breathing. Heavy or lengthy inhalation generates Yang energy, heavy or lengthy exhalation generates Yin energy, and holding one's breath balances both energies. So whenever you need a lift anytime, anywhere, you may inhale for fifteen seconds or fifteen counts, hold the breath for ten counts, and then exhale for five counts. To relax yourself anytime, anywhere, inhale for five counts, hold the breath for ten counts, and then exhale for fifteen counts. With these techniques, you can maintain a positive or calm demeanor in any negative situation. You are also free to extend the length of the inhalations or exhalations.

Brain Cleansing Exercises

The Brain Cleansing Exercises utilize the Turtle, Deer, and Crane breathing techniques to form the foundation upon which rests the Immortal Breathing. Without a firm foundation one cannot build a secure house which will be safe from the winds of disease and negative mental attitudes. So before beginning any of the breathing techniques, it is necessary to have practiced and to become proficient in combining the Deer, Crane, and Turtle Exercises.

We need to learn to relax not only the body, but also the mind. Our minds are hosts to tremendous amounts of unnecessary worry which produces undue tension and stress and may lead to acute and chronic diseases. The Brain Cleansing Breathing is a basic healing technique which works to wash away stress from within our minds. Negative thoughts are large obstacles which prevent healing from occurring within our system. Taoism holds that an idea or thought *is* reality. Thus a negative thought cultivates a negative condition within our physical bodies. By practicing the Brain Cleansing Exercises we gain a tool to empty the mind of all its useless thoughts, and bring it to a balanced state. If the mind is completely balanced, so also will be the body. If you feel sick, this is an imbalance, but even if you feel well, this too is an imbalance. Taoism asks one to feel nothing to either extreme but just to *act naturally in the middle way*. We must awaken to our native condition and become empty to the point where there is neither positive nor negative, neither hate nor love—just an openness. Thus we become something great and at peace with ourselves.

Empty yourself of everything.
Let the mind rest at peace.
The ten thousand things rise and fall while the Self watches their return.
They grow and flourish and then return to the source.
Returning to the source is stillness, which is the way of nature.
The way of nature is unchanging.
Knowing constancy is insight.
Not knowing constancy leads to disaster.
Knowing constancy, the mind is open.
With an open mind, you will be openhearted.
Being openhearted, you will act royally.
Being royal, you will attain the divine.
Being divine, you will be at one with the Tao.
Being at one with the Tao is eternal.
And though the body dies, the Tao will never pass away.

Tao Te Ching XVI

BRAIN CLEANSING I

Negative thoughts are large obstacles which prevent healing from occurring within the body. The Brain Cleansing I exercise helps to train the mind to become empty of negativities and to help it take on divine qualities. It will help one come into harmony with the natural laws of the universe, by enabling one to cast out the limiting concepts of wrong thinking and death and find the Tao, where there are no "isms" or dualistic thoughts, no desires, no diseases, but only complete peace.

1. Begin the Brain Cleansing I breathing exercise by assuming the Turtle sitting position. Sit with the back erect and with the hands

resting lightly on the knees. Clasp the thumbs securely between the fingers. In this manner you hold onto the energy in your hands so that it re-circulates back into the arms. Allow the eyes to remain closed throughout the exercise.

2. Now exhale all of the air from your lungs (without straining) as you assume the Turtle position with the head stretching upward and the shoulders down.

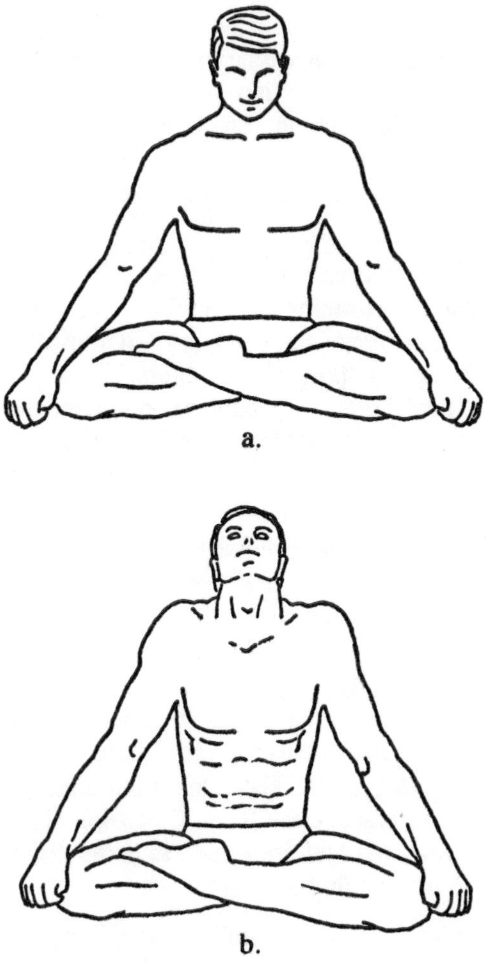

Figures 100a and 100b. Brain Cleansing I.

3. Next, gently tilt the head backward into the second Turtle position and slowly begin to inhale the breath. Try to feel that as the breath enters into the internal chambers of your body it carries with it a boiling steam, fire, or white smoke, and that it slowly begins to rise upward from the abdomen to the head. Feel the smoke fill the head completely.

4. When you have completed the inhalation (without straining), then straighten the head and begin to exhale in the first Turtle position. Feel the smoke, steam, or fire leave the body. Feel it carry out with it the worries, tensions, unnecessary thoughts, dishonesty, anger, depression, and ills of your mind and body. Feel the clearness and cleanness that is left behind. Then repeat the breathing sequence again as many times as you feel comfortable. However, try to maintain a minimum of seven inhalations and seven exhalations at each sitting.

NOTE A: It is important to remember to keep the anal muscles contracted while performing the exercise as this will lock the energy in the upper chambers of the body and will allow the energy and the smoke to rise up the spine, into the brain.

NOTE B: At first it may be difficult to coordinate the breathing with the sensations. But with determined and motivated practice, you will be able to clearly feel the smoke as it comes into and leaves your head. Also at first you may not be able to feel the clearness that is left behind, but with patient practice you will be able to develop a strong feeling of clarity. If the mind is clear, then your problems will be eighty percent eliminated.

BRAIN CLEANSING II

This exercise provides a marvelous stretch to the back, shoulders, and arms, as well as helping to balance your energy and relieve tension and fatigue from the body. It also keeps the mind alert and fresh.

It is beneficial to practice the Brain Cleansing II exercise at any time during the day when you feel tired, such as in the morning upon rising, at the office, or in the evening after work.

1. This exercise is performed while in a standing position (it may also be practiced from a prone position while lying on your back) with the feet slightly apart but parallel to each other. The hands are relaxed but

straight and are held at the sides of the body, and the head is in an upright position as in the first position of the Turtle Exercise.

2. Begin by exhaling the breath to completely empty the lungs.

3. Now drop the head back and begin to inhale slowly. As you inhale, expand the chest and bring the arms up away from the sides of your body so that you bring the hands together up over your head with the palms together. (Do not strain during any of these movements. If it is impossible to touch the hands together comfortably, simply raise the hands as far as they will go and stop there.) As you bring the arms up over the head, feel as if you are bringing in the active (yang) energy of the universe (or white smoke) into your lungs, body, and mind.

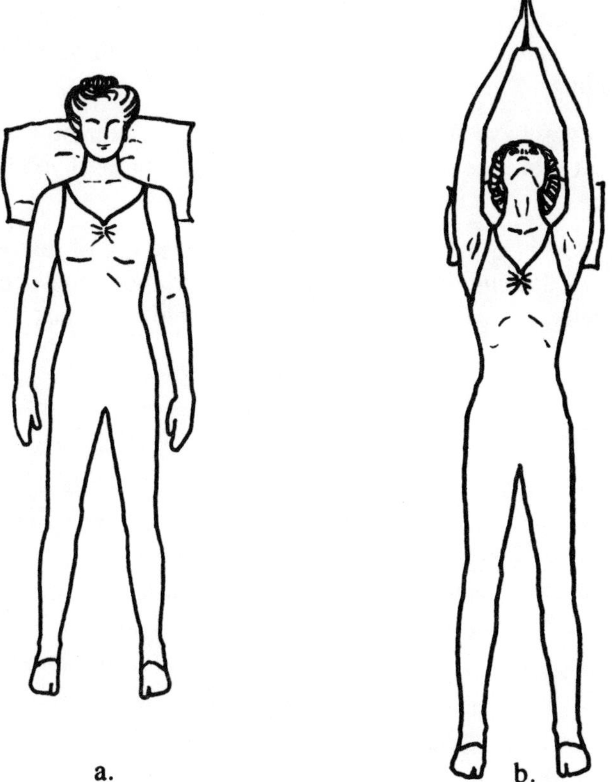

Figures 101a and 101b. Brain Cleansing II.

4. After you have inhaled a full breath, and while still keeping the arms held over your head, hold the breath in, lock your anal muscles and relax in this pose for as long as you can without strain. Feel as if the white smoke is coming up to completely penetrate every space inside the mind. Feel the energy circulate around within your body and your mind, knowing that it is beginning to wash away all of your negative thoughts.

5. Next, as you slowly begin to exhale, bring the head forward and separate the hands. Keeping the arms straight, move them back down to your sides. As your hands move in the downward arc, try to feel the passive (yin) energy from the earth (cool breezes) come into the arms through your fingers. This exercise is symbolic of embracing the entire universe so that one achieves a feeling of oneness from uniting the earthly passive energy with the active, heavenly energy. As you continue to exhale, feel the smoke leave, leaving behind a clean and clear feeling.

6. When you have finished exhaling, repeat the breathing and arm movement sequence a minimum of seven times or until you feel like stopping.

NOTE: It is refreshing to practice this exercise out of doors in the sunshine, gathering the fresh air into the body. As you perform the arm movements, feel as if you are reaching out to touch the clouds and the sky.

8

Immortal Breathing: Small and Large Heavenly Cycles

There are two special meridians surrounding the Seven Glands System. One is called the Jen-Mo Conception Meridian, and the other is called the Tu-Mo Governing Meridian. They are the only two meridians whose energy flows can be changed. If we change them we will bring about profound changes in the seven glands which will immortalize our bodies.

The seven glands of the human body are responsible for controlling all of the bodily functions. As mentioned earlier, they mutually balance and are interconnected with one another. They energize, recharge, and help circulate energy in the body, and may be likened to electrical transformers or generators or storehouses of energy within the human body. When the energy within the Seven Glands System is elevated to a higher frequency by the body, the entire body will be brought to a perfect or spiritual order.

Before undertaking the Immortal Breathing, it is necessary that you have already achieved sufficient expertise in the system of Internal Exercises so that the body is in a balanced state of health without any serious or chronic ailments. It is impossible to practice the final stages of the breathing exercises if there are any blockages in the meridian pathways. The Meridian Meditation and the other Internal Exercises are therefore necessary prerequisites for opening up the meridians and preparing the body for receiving the Immortal Breath.

The human body is an electrical system. It is capable of carrying a load of electricity through it only as strong as the resistance of the nerves and glands are to that electrical current. The stronger the body is physically, the greater the current load of electricity it will be able to handle.

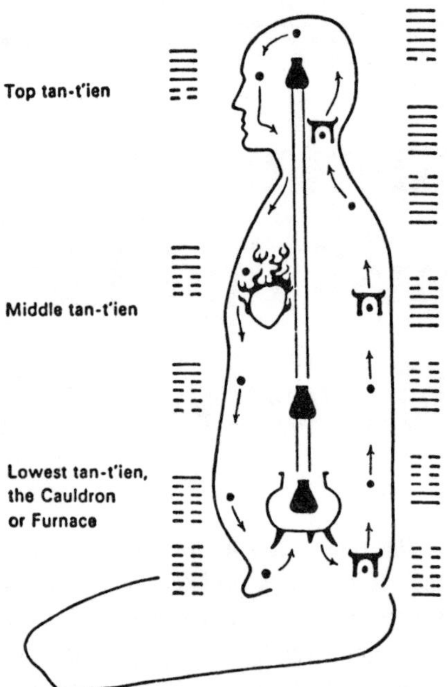

Figure 102. Schematic Representation of the Path of Energy Flow.

Immortal Breathing brings into the body very powerful levels of energy, and if the body is not sufficiently strong to handle it, the nerves and glands may "burn out" from an overload of energy. It has been said that many people who suffer from extreme mental conditions are that way only because they are unable to handle the energy levels flowing within their bodies. Unfortunately, if one experiences excessively high levels of energy over too long a period of time, irreversible damage may be done to the body. *Do not, therefore, regard the Immortal Breathing lightly.*

However, if you have followed the steps of the Internal Exercises and meditations conscientiously and have practiced the Crane, Turtle, and Deer Exercises so that you are proficient in them, you will be ready to begin the Immortal Breathing (the Immortal Breathing exercises are extensions of the Deer at a very, very elevated level).

This is the final stage of the Taoist system of Internal Exercises. Mastery of Immortal Breathing may require from one year to a lifetime of diligent practice. Letting the body raise its energy levels to higher frequencies is not something to be rushed. Promising miracles for a minimum of effort and time is a sin, for many lives can be ruined permanently, or "disintegrated into evil".

However, if impatience can be overcome, the rewards are indescribable. The spiritual eye of the practitioner is fully awakened, and he or she is raised to the level of the *Hsien*, or wise and immortal person. The *Hsien* is one who knows the secrets of the universe by being in complete union with the Tao, or God, exists perpetually, and has the power of the universe at his or her disposal. Is this not the true desire which lies in the hearts of all men? God has put this desire for spirituality in man—no other organism in the universe is so gifted—so that man may one day accompany him.

SMALL HEAVENLY CYCLE

This type of breathing is often called the "Self-Winding Wheel of the Law". When first practicing this type of breathing, one must use one's will power to initiate the cycle. However, there comes a time when the breathing becomes automatic and will continue on an involuntary basis. Thus, once the process has been initiated, it becomes something which, in a manner of speaking, becomes self-winding, irreversible and beyond one's control. In such a way the final stage of enlightenment comes not from something you are doing, but comes all of its own to you.

1. Sit with your spine and head held erect.

2. Grasp your thumbs inside your fingers and lay your hands lightly on your legs.

3. Begin to inhale slowly, without forcing your breath at any time. As you inhale, feel the breath come in through your nose and

descend through the Jen-Mo meridian into the abdominal cavity (stove) where the breath will be heated (transmuted) and energized.

4. When you have fully inhaled the breath, lock your anal sphincter muscles and pull your chin down onto your chest in a chin lock. These two movements prevent the energy from escaping the abdominal chamber and help to further energize the energy as it activates the sexual glands. Also, when you hold your breath, the blood vessels tend to constrict, thus raising the blood pressure. The chin lock helps to reverse this process and restore an equilibrium to the body.

5. With your breath held, and the anal and chin locks in place, begin to feel the energy in the stove cauldron (abdomen) beginning to rise upward along the back of the spinal column or Tu-Mo meridian.

6. As the energy travels upward, it moves through the seven houses (glands) in succession, entering first into the sexual glands where it makes a spiraling circular movement, and then passes upward and through the remaining six houses in similar wheel-like movements (see figure 103). The wheel rotations at each house serve to energize the house in which it occurs, as well as transform the energy into a higher order to be received by the next house. In this fashion each of the glands serves as transformer and generator for the energy of the body.

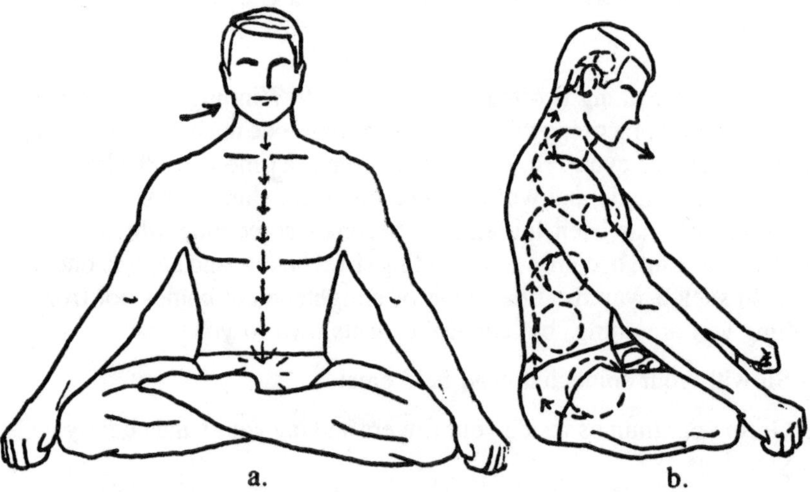

Figures 103a and 103b. Small Heavenly Cycle Sitting Pose.

7. When the energy reaches the level of the pineal gland, allow it to circulate there for a moment, and then release the anal and chin locks and slowly exhale the breath.

8. Begin the Small Heavenly Cycle again.

NOTE: At first you will want to hold the breath only for seven seconds, one second for each gland. As you become proficient in the breathing, hold the breath for longer periods of time. As the breath is held for longer periods, begin to make two or more loops around the houses for each period during which the breath is held. So the sequence would become: inhale the air into the abdomen through the Jen-Mo meridian; hold the breath and lock the chin and anal muscles; pass the energy up and through the Tu-Mo meridian into the sexual glands, adrenals, pancreas, thymus, thyroid, pituitary, and pineal glands, then back down the Jen-Mo, and so on until there is the need to exhale the breath. With practice the breath can be held for several minutes to several hours without feeling the need to breathe. When the seven houses have been sufficiently energized, the need to breathe disappears and one functions in a breathless state of immortality.

LARGE HEAVENLY CYCLE

The Large Heavenly Cycle, like the Small Heavenly Cycle, utilizes the breath and the seven basic houses (glands) of the body. The difference between the two techniques is that the Large Heavenly Cycle allows the energy to travel down the meridians of the legs and arms in addition to the central axial chamber of the body.

1. Begin in a seated position with the spine and head held erect.

2. Inhale the breath and allow it to pass through the Jen-Mo meridian in the front of the body to the abdominal cauldron (stove) where it will be fired up and energized.

3. After a full inhalation, perform the chin and anal lock, hold the breath, and allow the energy to circulate through the seven houses as described in the Small Heavenly Cycle.

4. When the energy has reached the pineal gland, allow it to descend again down the Jen-Mo meridian into the legs through the stomach, bladder, and gallbladder meridians which lie along the outside of the legs.

5. When the energy has reached your toes, bring it back up your legs through the spleen-pancreas, kidney, and liver meridians which lie along the inside of the legs.

6. Circulate the energy back up the spine along the Tu-Mo meridian and then allow it to descend down the arms through the lung, heart, and Heart Constrictor meridians which lie along the inside of each arm.

7. When the energy has reached the finger tips, allow the energy to pass back up the arms through the large intestine, small intestine, and Triple Heater meridians and bring it back into the Jen-Mo meridian and down to the abdominal cauldron.

8. This completes one Large Heavenly Cycle. You may now exhale the breath or continue to perform the breathing cycle until you feel the need to exhale the breath.

NOTE: At the beginning of your practice, hold your breath for seven seconds while feeling the energy around your body. With increased proficiency, increase the time to five minutes or more and perform as many rotations of the large cycle as possible, always ending the breath with the energy in the abdominal cauldron.

You may eventually reach the point where there is no need felt to inhale or exhale. It is at this level that the cells of the body have been transmuted through an alchemical process to where they are able to exist only on the energy which circulates throughout the universe, rather than on the grosser need for oxygen which is presently felt. It is at this point that the "normal" laws of time and space no longer bind the individual to this body or earth, and one has entered into the eternal nature of the universe.

PART IV

BEGINNING ANEW:

FINDING PROBLEMS, SOLVING PROBLEMS

9

Taoist Healing Prescriptions

The Internal Exercises may be divided into four distinct categories: 1) general and regular health maintenance exercises; 2) specific healing exercises for individual organs or parts of the body; 3) breathing exercises; and 4) meditative and contemplative techniques. In addition, there are healing prescriptions which combine several of the Internal Exercise techniques and are used when treating a specific disease or ailment.

The general health maintenance exercises are to be practiced on a daily basis for a minimum of three months.Then one should continue to practice the Deer, Crane, and Turtle daily, and use the other exercises on a schedule of alternate days or weeks so as to build the body to its maximum level of health. After about three months one should be able to feel the flow of energy in the body as one practices these exercises. When one can perceive this subtle flow of energy or life force (Chi) within the body, then it will be time to begin practicing the Meridian Meditation techniques. To properly learn the contemplative exercises takes between one and ten years.

Develop patience in your practice and you will escape "Disintegration into Evil" and be rewarded generously. Practicing the Taoist Internal Exercises is like venturing into a dark cave and discovering a treasure which has been lying there for years awaiting its discovery. Upon returning to the sunlight, that treasure will sparkle magnificently. The treasure is your health and the Taoists feel that perfect health is our birthright.

You may find from time to time that you will go through periods when you are unable to perform your exercises (because of location, family crisis, etc.) If you have become genuinely interested and are able to see the benefits you will have accrued from doing the Internal Exercises up to that point, have faith that you will return and begin again where you left off. The Internal Exercise system is to be practiced throughout your lifetime. Therefore, minor periods when one does not practice them will be insignificant if one follows them for the bulk of one's lifetime.

The constitutions of some people upon beginning the Internal Exercises may be very weak, or there may be chronic problems which have been developing over the years. Even if one practices the exercises, whether because of poor diet or an excess of stress in one's daily life or through injury, one may acquire diseases or problems of health, such as heart disease, obesity, or lower back pain. Included in the system of Internal Exercises, therefore, are techniques designed to deal with specific problems of the body. These are prescribed on an individual level, and are to be practiced until the disease, pain, or problem disappears entirely. They are to be practiced in conjunction with the other general health maintenance exercises.

Included in this chapter are also healing prescriptions or combinations of several Internal Exercises which, when practiced together, aid the natural healing processes in certain states of discomfort or disease, such as migraine headaches, high blood pressure, or hemorrhoids.

General Health Maintenance Schedule

Upon waking in the morning:

Toe Wiggling and Body Stretching
Internal Organ Relaxation
Head Rubbing Exercise
Eye Exercises
Nose Exercise
Beating the Heavenly Drum

Mouth Exercises
Face Rubbing Exercise
Kidney Exercise
Liver Exercise
Solar Plexus Exercise
Meridian Massage
Deer Exercise
Crane Exercise
Turtle Exercise

Regular Health Maintenance

To be done daily throughout one's life:

Five Animal Exercises
Eight Directional Exercises
Twelve Zodiac Exercises
Twelve Nerve Exercises

Meditation

Upon feeling the subtle energy flow in the body, one may begin practicing the meditation:

Meridian Meditation

Only after mastering the Meridian Meditation should one begin to practice the Immortal Breathing techniques.

Specific Healing Exercises

These may be practiced in conjunction with the general health maintenance exercises or just for correcting specific ailments.

Weight Reduction Exercise
Lower Back Exercises
Stomach Healing Exercise
Heart Exercises
Abdominal Strengthening Exercise
Lung Exercise
Lower Body and Sexual Glands Exercise
Techniques for Relieving Pain
Hand, Arm, and Upper Body Exercises

Sun Worship Exercise
Eye Exercises
Internal Organ Relaxation
Relaxation exercises

Breathing Exercises Include:

Crane Exercise
Heart Healing Exercise
Reverse Crane I
Reverse Crane II
Bone Breathing
Brain Cleansing I
Brain Cleansing II
Immortal Breathing:
  Small Heavenly Cycle
  Large Heavenly Cycle

HEALING PRESCRIPTIONS

Arthritis, Rheumatism, Bursitis, Tennis Elbow:

Turtle
Crane
Deer
Arm stimulating exercises (for tennis elbow, rub until you feel the arm become hot around the elbow—feel the heat in the elbow)
Leg stimulating exercises
Arm and Hand Pressing Exercise (for bursitis or arthritis in arms or hands)
Techniques for Relieving Pain

Asthma:

Crane, Turtle, Deer—all practiced together
Lung Exercise
Liver Exercise (soothes and strengthens the nerves)

Back Pain:

Lower Back Exercises
Kidney Exercise

Beauty and Fitness (rejuvenation)

Deer, Crane, Turtle
Eye Exercises (for wrinkles)
Gum Pressure Exercise
Tongue and Saliva Exercise
Beating the Heavenly Drum
Teeth Clicking Exercise
Weight Reduction Exercise
Solar Plexus Exercise
Head Rubbing Exercise
Breathing exercises

Blood Pressure—High:

Crane, Turtle (avoid Deer until pressure falls to normal)
Brain Cleansing I
Toe wiggling exercise

Blood Pressure—Low:

Deer, Turtle (avoid Crane until pressure comes up)
Brain Cleansing II
Toe wiggling exercise

Bronchitis (throat pains):

Lung exercises
Meridian Massage (especially downward along lung meridian)
Solar Plexus Exercise

Cancer,

Bone:

Kidney Exercise
Lower Back Exercises
Liver Exercise

Prevention:

Crane, Turtle, Deer
Arm stimulating exercises
Kneading shoulder muscles (releases tension and stress and opens meridians which may be blocked)

Cellulite:

Leg stimulating exercises (rub downward on outside only)
Lower Body and Sexual Glands Exercise

Common Cold (sneezing, coughing, sinus headache):

Internal Organ Relaxation (brings blood into head and lungs to fight head cold)
Nose Exercise (for sinus)
Head Rubbing Exercise (pressing points behind head for headache and tension)
Pressing on either side of the throat on stomach meridian points (this may cause you to cough at first, but it will eventually stop the coughing)
Meridian Massage (rubbing downward along the lung meridian for temporary relief of cold symptoms and lung congestion)

Concentration Problems:

Five Animal Exercises
Concentration Exercise

Constipation:

Crane breathing
Solar Plexus Exercise
Twelve Zodiac Exercises

Diabetes:

Liver and pancreas rubbing exercise
Leg stimulating exercises (especially upward rubbing on the inside of the leg to bring energy into the body)
Deer Exercise

Tongue and Saliva Exercise (for relief of symptoms of thirst caused by diabetes)

Diarrhea:

Deer
Leg stimulating exercises (upward rubbing on inside of leg only)
Solar Plexus Exercise

Dizziness (vertigo, nerve imbalance):

Bone Breathing
Ear Exercise
Brain Cleansing II
Turtle, Crane

Emphysema:

See *Asthma*

Eye Problems (glaucoma, cataract, near- and far-sightedness, etc.):

Eye Exercises

Female Problems:

Deer
Kidney Exercise
Leg stimulating exercise (on the inside of legs only)
Solar Plexus Exercise

Headache:

Bone Breathing
Eye Exercises
Nose Exercise
Standing Crane
Brain Cleansing II
Head Rubbing Exercise (rub points behind head)

Hearing Problems:

Ear Exercise

Heart Problems:

Heart Exercises

Hepatitis (liver problems):

Liver Exercise

Hemorrhoids:

Deer Exercise (squeezing anal muscles)
Sun Worship Exercise

Impotence (premature ejaculation):

Deer
Brain Cleansing I
Sexual gland exercise

Insomnia

Toe wiggling exercise
Crane breathing
Bone Breathing
Solar Plexus Exercise

Kidney Problems:

Kidney Exercise
Deer
Leg stimulating exercise (upward on the inside only)

Menstrual Problems:

See *Female Problems*

Nerve Problems (numbness and paralysis):

See also *Liver Problems*
Crane, Deer, Turtle
Liver Exercise
Rubbing local area until warm to bring in fresh blood and energy
Twelve Nerve Exercises

Obesity:

Weight Reduction Exercise
Solar Plexus Exercise

Overacidity:

Crane
Liver Exercise (calms and balances stomach)

Pneumonia:

Crane breathing (to help rest lungs, very slowly)
Rubbing downward along lung meridian (for temporary relief)

Prostate Problems:

Deer

Refreshing Yourself:

Five Animal Exercises
Eight Directional Exercises
Twelve Nerve Exercises
Deer, Crane, Turtle
Reverse Crane I
Reverse Crane II
Bone Breathing
Energizing and Relaxing Breathing Exercises
Internal Organ Relaxation
Eye Exercises

Sciatica:

Leg stimulating exercise
Lower Back Exercises
Lower Body and Sexual Glands Exercise

Stomach Problems (ulcers, pain, vomiting):

See also *Diarrhea*
Crane
Solar Plexus Exercise

Stomach Healing Exercise

Stomach Problems (nausea from hypoglycemia):

Liver Exercise
Rubbing across pancreas

Tennis Elbow:

See *Arthritis*

Teeth and Gum Problems:

Mouth Exercises

Thyroid Problems:

Thyroid Exercise

Tonsilitis:

Turtle
Throat rubbing

Tuberculosis:

Crane

Coughing complications:

Rubbing down inside of arms
Throat rubbing

Sweating complications:

Toe wiggling exercise (calming)

Diarrhea complications:

Solar Plexus Exercise
Crane, Deer

Ulcer:

See *Stomach Problems* and *Nerve Problems*

Vomiting:

Crane
Stomach exercises

All illnesses:

Five Animal Exercises
Eight Directional Exercises
Twelve Zodiac Exercises
Twelve Nerve Exercises

Conclusion

When thinking about integrating the system of Internal Exercises (or the Tao of Revitalization) into our daily lives, it is important to keep in mind the ancient Taoist proverb which states simply: "If you do external exercises, you *must* do internal exercises". External exercises expend energy without replacing it, and therefore we feel a need to rest after strenuous physical activity. On the other hand, Internal Exercises work to conserve and build up our energy. The proverb continues: "If you do internal exercises, you may forget to practice external exercises"—because one benefits completely through the practice of Internal Exercises.

This is not to imply that one should not practice external exercises such as tennis, running, or golf. The Taoists were only recognizing the fact that, by themselves, external exercises are incomplete and need to be balanced by the addition of these simple techniques for rebalancing and supplanting the loss of energy incurred through external exercises.

The Internal Exercises energize, train, and strengthen the internal organs and tissues so they may become strong and healthy. When the internal body and mind is strong, we will lack the opportunity to become diseased. The beauty of the Internal Exercises is that they are very easy to practice. No matter where you are or what time it is, it is possible to practice these simple techniques: when you are driving along in your car, do the Deer Exercise by squeezing the sphincter muscles. Nothing could be simpler or easier to practice; no special equipment is needed and no one else need know what you are doing!

In addition, Internal Exercises encourage the circulatory system without speeding up the heart rate. All the exercises are done slowly, without effort. You see, the number of times our heart beats during our lifetime indicates the length of our life. We do not want the heart to wear out prematurely. The heart rate does not increase during the practice of these exercises and, yet, through their practice the heart rate actually slows down. We are therefore able to increase our life expectancy as the ancient Taoists wished.

Oftentimes, people who practice external exercises become involved in a subtle, yet destructive cycle. External exercises work to train the muscular system. Vigorous exercise often stimulates the appetite and the person in training ends up eating more than he or she would otherwise. All goes well until the person stops exercising, and then all the muscles which have been built up turn to fatty tissues. *This does not occur through the practice of the Internal Exercises.* They work to control the size and tightness of the muscles and other tissues without encouraging the appetite. As a matter of fact, many report that the Turtle Exercise actually decreases their appetite.

The ancient Taoists recognized that the Internal Exercises follow natural laws in working to fulfill their final purpose. Will power is not necessary to practice these exercises, for one is not interested in making impossible things occur, only in doing what is possible. By practicing the Internal Exercises, one forgets oneself and the ego becomes smaller, while the spirit or god within becomes larger.

There are four kingdoms in the universe. The first, or Vegetable Kingdom, has no purpose other than to exist and grow; plants and one-celled organisms have no mind of their own. The second, or Animal Kingdom, has mind and soul, but lacks a spirit and therefore has no purpose other than to propagate itself. The third realm, the Human Kingdom, has mind, soul, and spirit. If we ask why man has religion, we realize that man is not content with his situation as it is. Animals do not seem to care about their situation, but man does. He has a higher purpose than merely to exist. This is exemplified in man's pursuit of his material life—he always wants something more than he has. We also have a desire to improve ourselves. Why? Because we have a spiritual need to improve ourselves into the Kingdom of God. To be religious means to find a way to get into the divine Kingdom of God—the fourth realm of this universe—to become immortal. The ancient Taoists recognized this primal urge of mankind and through their knowledge of the natural laws perfected this system of Internal Exercises as a means whereby—with daily practice—man could realize his birthright, his divine self. The system of Internal Exercises is meant to provide each of us with the opportunity to unify our bodies with our minds and our spiritual selves. Only then can we realize the Tao, our true immortality, and enter into the Kingdom of God.

Index

Index